The New Nurse Educator

Deborah Dolan Hunt, PhD, RN, is Assistant Professor of Nursing at The College of New Rochelle where she serves on several internal committees including the School of Nursing Team Committee, the Undergraduate Committee, the Program Effectiveness Committee, and several "external" college committees including the Council of Faculty and the Academic Affairs Committee. She has also served as a mentor, preceptor, and role model to several graduate students during their capstone class in nursing education. She is the co-founder and co-director of the Nurse Advocacy Forum at The College of New Rochelle. She is on the regional editorial advisory board at Advance for Nurses Northeast Region. She has also served as a peer reviewer for several journals and book chapters and has been published in *American Nurse Today, Nurse Spectrum, Nursing Made Incredibly Easy,* and *Advance for Nurses.* Dr. Hunt is currently serving as one of the nurse co-leads for the New York State Future of Nurses Action Coalition in the Northern Metropolitan region of New York. She is a member of Community Board No. 10 in the Bronx and the chairperson of its Health and Human Services Committee. She was also appointed by Councilman James Vacca to serve as a member of the Aging Improvement District Advisory Board. She was recently accepted as a fellow in the New York Academy of Medicine. Prior to her current role in academia, Dr. Hunt spent ten years in Staff Development. She is a member of Sigma Theta Tau International Honor Society of Nursing and received the Zeta Omega research award for her doctoral dissertation and was the Sigma Theta Tau's Zeta Omega Scholar from 2010–2011. She earned her PhD from Adelphi University, her MS degree in Nursing Administration from The College of New Rochelle, and a BSN from Mercy College. She has presented both locally and internationally and recently received the Faculty Fund Award at The College of New Rochelle to conduct a phenomenological study with her colleague and mentor, Dr. Connie Vance.

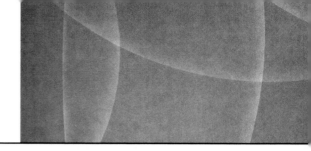

The New Nurse Educator

Mastering Academe

Deborah Dolan Hunt, PhD, RN

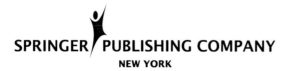

SPRINGER PUBLISHING COMPANY

NEW YORK

Springer Publishing Company, LLC
11 West 42nd Street
New York, NY 10036
www.springerpub.com

Acquisitions Editor: Margaret Zuccarini
Composition: diacriTech

ISBN: 978-0-8261-0641-4
E-book ISBN: 978-0-8261-0642-1

15 /6

The author and the publisher of this Work have made every effort to use sources believed to be reliable to provide information that is accurate and compatible with the standards generally accepted at the time of publication. Because medical science is continually advancing, our knowledge base continues to expand. Therefore, as new information becomes available, changes in procedures become necessary. We recommend that the reader always consult current research and specific institutional policies before performing any clinical procedure. The author and publisher shall not be liable for any special, consequential, or exemplary damages resulting, in whole or in part, from the readers' use of, or reliance on, the information contained in this book. The publisher has no responsibility for the persistence or accuracy of URLs for external or third-party Internet Web sites referred to in this publication and does not guarantee that any content on such Web sites is, or will remain, accurate or appropriate.

Library of Congress Cataloging-in-Publication Data is available from the Library of Congress.

Printed in the United States of America by Gasch Printing.

This book is dedicated with love and gratitude to my parents Patrick and Rita Dolan, my husband Brian, and my children Brian, Meaghan, and John, to Jessica, and to all my family, friends, colleagues, and students.

It is also dedicated to my teachers and mentors and to all the past, current, and future nurse educators. May we always find joy in preparing and mentoring the nurses of tomorrow!

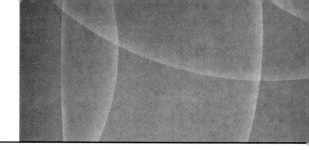

Contents

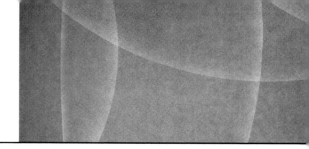

Foreword

"You have brains in your head. You have feet in your shoes. You can steer yourself any direction you choose. You're on your own. And you know what you know. And YOU are the one who'll decide where to go"

—Dr. Seuss, *Oh, the Places You'll Go!*

I wish I had this book available to me when I transitioned from the position of clinical educator to the position of academic educator. I was so overwhelmed when I assumed my first faculty position that I did not know enough to know what to ask! Every aspect of academia was new for me and I did not know what direction to go in first. On my first day as "professor," I was handed the faculty handbook. It was a necessary source of information that primed me about my role as novice educator but did not include the details required to move seamlessly, comfortably, and competently from novice to expert educator. What I really desired was to know what was "between the lines." The topics in this book, ranging from how to prepare course materials to how to develop a professional educational portfolio for tenure consideration, filled in those blanks. Read in entirety, the chapters are structured to create a road map for success in the academic or clinical educator role. Lack of information required to complete a basic project such as creating reliable and valid examinations or utilizing a learning management system to its potential can make a simple task appear monumental. The depth and breadth of information and resources in this book provide resources valuable not only for the novice educator but also resources to complement specific aspects of the expert educator's role.

The value of this book is that it was written by a nurse educator who presents a view of the journey from clinical educator to academic educator that remains grounded in the demands being made on nurses and nurse educators in the 21st century. Wisdom garnered from Dr. Hunt's personal journey is supported with scholarly evidence to assist a novice or more experienced educator, to navigate and balance the complex and often competing demands of teaching, scholarship, and service. Content clearly reflects The National League for Nursing and American Association of Colleges of Nursing competencies and, while broad in scope as well as extensive in detail, is written in an engaging narrative style enhanced by timely references and reflective insights from individual nurse educators in a wide variety of settings.

Dr. Hunt has been my colleague for many years and I am honored to prepare this introduction. We shared office space when she first came to the school of nursing as a clinical instructor and novice academic educator. I am now in awe of the way Dr. Hunt has interwoven her personal journey with evidence-based references and scholarly insights.

Lynda Shand RN, PhD, MA, BSN, CNE, CHPN,
Associate Professor,
Coordinator, Education Track,
Master's Program,
The College of New Rochelle School of Nursing,
New Rochelle, New York.

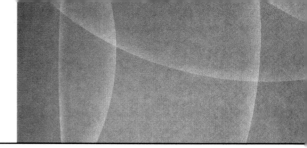

Preface

My goal in writing this book was to offer new and aspiring nurse educators a hands-on role development guide to use throughout their journey as nurse educators.

I feel this book is especially significant in light of the nurse faculty shortage and the Institute of Medicine's Future of Nursing Report, which calls for the advanced education for all nurses. I hope that experienced faculty may also find this book helpful, especially as they become mentors to new nurse educators.

When I transitioned from service to academe, I was filled with excitement and some trepidation about functioning within this new role. I believed the transition would be challenging, but since I had spent so many years in Staff Development I thought it would be fairly smooth. Boy, was I in for a surprise! I soon realized I was back in Patricia Benner's "novice stage" and had to figure out how to transition once again to the "expert stage"—I even wrote an article for *Advance for Nurses* called "Still a Novice After Twenty Years."

I remember my friend and colleague, Kathleen Cino, who was one of my first mentors at The College of New Rochelle (CNR), shared the following with me: "At the beginning of the semester, you get on the train and you don't stop until the end of the semester"—it certainly felt like that. There was so much to do and so little time to do it. Developing the syllabus, outlines, lesson plans, assignments, exams, and trying to teach in a creative way were monumental tasks. Sometimes I would look out at the perplexed faces of my students and want to run out of the classroom. But at some point along the way, I found my comfort zone, and now I look at faces that really are interested in hearing what I have to say. Recognizing this turning point was a great moment for me, a novice educator. At the end of that semester, when students sent me notes actually thanking me, it was an incredible joy! I knew then that academe had chosen me just as I had chosen academe.

However, there were still hurdles to overcome. When I was told I had to advise 30 students, I nearly fainted. Then there were meetings and office hours and a myriad of students' issues and other assorted meetings. In the midst of all this, I was applying to graduate school. I also did not really understand the requirements for teaching, scholarship, and service, especially in relation to tenure and promotion. Lucky for me, the faculty at CNR took me under their collective wing and each one helped me in a different way. I have always been an avid reader and read everything I could find about being a nurse educator; although I found many wonderful resources, I was looking for something more hands on and this is what prompted me to write this book.

I thought back to my experience and knew that if I had not had the caring and generous faculty colleagues at CNR I might not have been successful. With that in mind, I developed this book under the triad of teaching, scholarship, and service. Throughout the chapters I have tried to share practical advice and examples of tools that helped me along the way. Part I contains an overview of the world of education and includes topics such as roles and responsibilities, educational preparation requirements, how to utilize past nursing experiences in this new role, the interview process, and ways to "test the waters." The focus of Part II is on the teaching role: Chapters in this section relate to all aspects of teaching, including learning styles, curriculum development, professional ethics, and theoretical frameworks in addition to legal issues for the nurse educator. Part III is on the role of a faculty member and includes topics such as tenure and promotion, collegiality, service, leadership, and mentoring. Part IV is on scholarship and includes topics such as writing for publication, research, and scholarly activities. The final section, Part V, is on special considerations and includes cultural diversity, students with disabilities, and reflective journaling.

Each chapter includes learning objectives and review questions along with suggested assignments that are intended to assist the teacher and student in professional role development. Additionally, the text prepares students for the academic interview process and includes sample CVs, patient education handouts, course objectives, and additional resources. Included in many of the chapters are reflections and advice from new and seasoned nurse educators, a well-known and highly respected nurse theorist, and a national nurse leader. Additionally, the mentoring chapter has been written by my friend, colleague, and mentor, Dr. Connie Vance, who is a recognized expert in the field of mentoring.

Although a good portion of this book relates to academic teaching, it applies to hospital-based educators as well. I hope that you will find as much joy and satisfaction in teaching as I have. I am happy to say that my journey from clinician to educator has been incredible, but it is also one of the most rewarding roles of my career. I have not quite reached the "expert stage" but have a plan on how to get there through the triad of teaching, scholarship, and service. The transition from the role of nurse educator in service to the role of nurse educator in academe is a challenging one. I hope this book will serve as a valuable guide on how to make that transition effectively.

Deborah Dolan Hunt

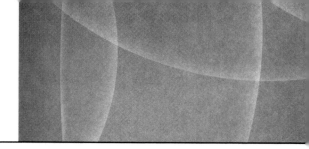

Acknowledgments

There are several individuals I would like to acknowledge. This book would not have been possible without the support and encouragement of Margaret Zuccarini, Publisher at Springer Publishing Company. Her sage advice was invaluable throughout this entire project. Christina Ferraro and Chris Teja, Assistant Editors, were also extremely helpful as I was completing this book. Joanne Jay was also extremely supportive in the final stages of this project. Dr. Connie Vance, my friend and mentor, encouraged me along the way and generously authored the chapter on mentoring. I would like to acknowledge Dr. Mimi Donius, Dr. Mary McGuinness, and Dr. Dorothy Escribano, and the rest of the faculty, administration, and staff at CNR, who are always there to encourage and support me on all of my projects, and Dr. Jane White who helped me to develop as a scholar and a writer. I would like to recognize all of my teachers, nurse colleagues, nursing students, and patients who were the real impetus for this book. A special note of gratitude to all of the nursing academic professionals who so generously contributed to this book: Dr. Geraldine (Polly) Bednash, Dr. Rhonda Brogdon, Dr. Mimi Donius, Dr. Terry Fulmer, Dr. Marianne Jeffreys, Dr. Carole Kenner, Dr. Donna Carol Maheady, Ms. Vicki Martin, Dr. Deborah Witt Sherman, Dr. Jean Watson, Dr. Ruth Wittmann-Price, Dr. Launette Woolforde, Dr. Lynda Shand. I would like to recognize my colleagues and students at The College of New Rochelle who have helped me learn how to become a proficient nurse educator. I have been blessed to have so many wonderful colleagues and students and I have learned something valuable from each and every one of them. I would also like to acknowledge the following authors for granting me permission to include their work in this book: Dr. Marianne Jeffreys, Dr. Madeleine Leininger, and Ms. Cohen.

Lastly, I would like to acknowledge my family and friends who are always there to support me in my personal and professional journeys.

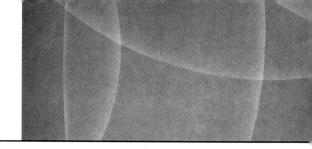

Contributors

Geraldine (Polly) Bednash, PhD, RN, FAAN
CEO and Executive Director, American Association of Colleges of Nursing (AACN), Washington, DC

Rhonda Brogdon, DNP, MSN, MBA, RN
Assistant Professor of Nursing, Francis Marion University, Florence, South Carolina

Mary Alice Higgins Donius, EdD, RN
Dean, The College of New Rochelle School of Nursing, New Rochelle, New York

Terry T. Fulmer, PhD, RN, FAAN
Dean, Bouve College of Health Sciences, Northeastern University, Boston, Massachusetts

Marianne R. Jeffreys, EdD, RN
Professor, Nursing, The City University of New York (CUNY) Graduate College, New York, New York
Professor, Nursing, CUNY College of Staten Island, Staten Island, New York

Carole Kenner, PhD, RNC-NIC, FAAN
Dean and Professor, Northeastern University School of Nursing, Associate Dean, Bouvé College of Health Science, Northeastern University, Boston, Massachusetts

Donna Carol Maheady, EdD, ARNP
Founder and President, ExceptionalNurse.com
Adjunct Faculty, Christine E. Lynn College of Nursing, Florida Atlantic University, Boca, Raton, Florida

Vicki Martin, MSN, RN
Instructor, Department of Nursing, Francis Marion University, Florence, South Carolina

Deborah Witt Sherman, PhD, CRNP, ANP-BC, ACHPN, FAAN
Professor, Co-Director of the Center for Excellence in Palliative Care Research, University of Maryland, School of Nursing, Baltimore, Maryland

Connie Vance, EdD, RN, FAAN
Professor, College of New Rochelle School of Nursing, New Rochelle, New York

Jean Watson, PhD, RN, AHN-BC, FAAN
Distinguished Professor/Endowed Chair in Caring Science, Founder, Watson Caring Science Institute, University of Colorado, Boulder, Colorado

Ruth A. Wittmann-Price, PhD, RN, CNS, CNE
Professor and Chair, Department of Nursing, Francis Marion University, Florence, South Carolina

Launette Woolforde, EdD(c), DNP, RN-BC
Corporate Director, Nursing Education, North Shore-LIJ Health System, Manhassett, New York

PART I

Introduction to the World of Nursing Education

CHAPTER 1

Educator Roles and Responsibilities: Teaching, Service, and Scholarship

"Tell me and I forget. Show me and I remember.
Involve me and I understand."

—CHINESE PROVERB

OBJECTIVES

After reading this chapter, the reader will be able to
- Discuss current trends for nurse faculty
- Compare and contrast roles of the nurse educator in service and academia
- Discuss requirements for nurse faculty in academia
- Discuss teaching, scholarship, and service expectations
- Identify key components of academic integrity and professional ethics

CURRENT STATISTICS AND PROJECTIONS FOR FACULTY

Historically, the role of the nurse educator can be traced back to Florence Nightingale, who has been identified as the "founder of modern nursing" and the "ultimate nurse educator" (Bastable, 2003, p. 4). Nightingale developed the first school of nursing in England in 1860. It was named the Nightingale School for Nurses and its mission was to train nurses to teach, and to care for the sick and the poor both in hospitals and in patients' homes (Neeb, 2006). In 1873, the Bellevue Training School for Nurses was established in New York City. This school along with several others established in the United States at that time followed the educational principles set forth by Florence Nightingale (McCloskey & Grace, 1981). Today there are over 3000 nursing programs in the United States (Gilbert, 2003) with approximately 1500 basic nursing education programs. Most of these programs still identify with the original mission of Florence Nightingale. These programs include more than 800 associate degree programs (Mahaffey, 2002), approximately 674 baccalaureate programs (Amos, 2005), and over 1000 graduate programs (Grad

Schools.com, 2010). Even with this number of programs, in 2008 there were 48,948 qualified applicants who were turned away due to a shortage of faculty, budgetary constraints, lack of preceptors, and inadequate clinical sites (American Association of Colleges of Nursing [AACN], 2010). Currently, there are approximately 41,605 to 48,666 nurse educators/faculty in the United States. While the number of faculty has increased from 2002–2006 there is still a faculty vacancy rate of 5.6% in associate degree programs and a vacancy rate of 7.9% in baccalaureate and higher education programs (Siela, Keller, & Connolly, 2008). The shortage of faculty is expected to grow with current projections of a 12% shortfall of nursing faculty within the next five years. The faculty shortage is related to salary and educational requirements and is a contributing factor in the current nursing shortage. In the United States the current RN vacancy rate is 8.1% with predictions of a shortage of 260,000 nurses by the year 2025 (AACN, 2010). Therefore, it is imperative to address the faculty shortage in order to increase enrollment in nursing schools around the country. The academic role is rewarding and challenging and this is the perfect time to transition to a faculty position. If teaching is your passion, there are several ways for you to become a nurse educator. The role of the nurse educator in service is quite different from the role in academia, but both are very rewarding.

EDUCATOR ROLES

Health Care Organizations/Service

All nurses have some responsibility to provide education throughout their careers. This is most often in the form of providing patient education to patients, families, and significant others. Most nurse generalist programs offer a basic review and application of the principles of education and patient teaching, thus providing the nurse with the foundation required of all nurse educators. Another informal way to teach is in the role of a preceptor or peer mentor for new graduates and newly hired staff. A preceptor development program will usually be offered to nurses who volunteer to become a preceptor. Often this is the impetus for a nurse to decide on the path to becoming a nurse educator.

Many nurse educators begin their professional development in a health care agency setting in roles such as an in-service educator, patient educator, clinical specialist, or staff development coordinator. This foundational experience in education is most often the stimulus for a nurse to enter into a more formal teaching role. The titles may vary but the nurse educator role in the hospital setting is similar. The roles and responsibilities of the hospital-based educator most often include staff orientation, continuing education, and facilitating clinical competencies of nursing staff. Some organizations have an entire department of nurse educators, while others have only one nurse educator. If an organization has an education department, there is usually a high degree of specialization with some educators responsible for orientation and others responsible for unit-based education. In a smaller organization there may be one or two nurse educators who share the teaching responsibilities. The focus of this type of education is driven by regulatory agencies, standards of care and practice, technology, quality and safety, clinical competence, nursing practice, performance improvement, patient satisfaction, ethical issues, and legal guidelines. Hence, the hospital-based educator must be knowledgeable about all of these issues in addition to teaching and learning theories of the adult learner. The nurse educator in the academic setting must also be knowledgeable in these areas but has some additional responsibilities and requirements and the academic setting is quite different from the health care setting.

Academe

The role of nurse educator in the academic setting is similar to the hospital-based educator yet also quite different. Teaching roles in academia include: clinical instructor, adjunct faculty, instructor of nursing, lecturer, assistant professor, associate professor, and full professor. Academic settings include the associate degree or diploma program, the baccalaureate degree program, the master's degree program, and the doctoral degree program. In each of these settings the roles and expectations will vary but the actual teaching role will always be at the forefront. These educational institutions develop role expectations and teaching requirements based on the mission, philosophy, and identity of the college, the State Board of Education, and standards of accreditation agencies such as the Middle States. The two accreditation agencies for nurse education programs are the Commission on Collegiate Nursing Education (CCNE) for baccalaureate, graduate, and residency programs in nursing, and the National League for Nurses (NLN) for associate degree programs in nursing.

Past nursing experience and level of education will dictate what setting is appropriate for new nurse faculty. For example, a nurse with a strong background in maternal child who has a master's degree will be eligible to teach maternal child health theory and clinical courses in an associate degree program. They may also be eligible to teach in a baccalaureate program as an adjunct or full-time tenure track faculty if they are planning to enroll in a doctoral degree program.

Full-time educators are often in a tenure track position. The faculty member is given a certain amount of time in years to develop and document evidence of excellence in teaching, service, and scholarship. Nurse faculty should be well versed in the tenure requirements for their organization and develop a plan to meet these standards. The Association of University Professors (AAUP) develops standards to protect academic freedom. They have been in existence for the past 90 years and are considered the voice of authority in this topic. In 1940, the AAUP in collaboration with the American Association of Colleges and Universities agreed upon a restatement of the principles developed in 1925 and published the 1940 *Statement of Principles on Academic Freedom and Tenure*. The complete document may be accessed at www.aaup.com. The basic tenets of this statement include: freedom of inquiry by teachers and students, freedom to research, freedom to teach controversial subject matter as long as it relates to the course, and freedom to write or speak without censure of discipline. However, the faculty member must exercise sound judgment in teaching and scholarship (AAUP, 2010). As the AAUP's core policy statement argues, "Institutions of higher education are conducted for the common good and not to further the interest of either the individual teacher or the institution as a whole. The common good depends upon the free search for truth and its free exposition" (1940 *Statement of Principles on Academic Freedom and Tenure*; AAUP, 2010, para. 1). Tenure is viewed as a means to protect academic freedom of faculty. "Tenure briefly stated, is an arrangement whereby faculty members, after successful completion of a period of probationary service, can be dismissed only for adequate cause or other possible circumstances and only after a hearing before a faculty committee" (AAUP, 2010). Every college and university has specific guidelines for tenure and promotion and new nurse faculty should review these carefully as they will be expected to maintain and present a portfolio of their accomplishments.

Many full-time nurse faculty begin their transition into the world of academia as clinical instructors or adjunct faculty. It is a wonderful way to "test the waters" and discover if an academic setting is the right fit. Most nursing schools utilize adjunct clinical faculty who have excellent clinical experience and are master's prepared. This foundational experience in education is most often the stimulus for a nurse to enter into a more formal teaching role.

TEACHING, SERVICE, AND SCHOLARSHIP

Teaching, service, and scholarship are the three areas where all faculty must excel. Just like reading, writing, and arithmetic are vital to the success of every student, teaching, learning, and scholarship are vital to the success of every faculty member. The importance of these collectively and individually varies according to the Carnegie classification of an institution. For example, at the university level the scholarship of teaching is still the main work of the nurse educator, but scholarship in the form of funded research is weighted more heavily. For example, many faculty appointments at the university level require the applicant to have a history of funded research endeavors. Conversely, at the college level research is expected but not at the same level as a university setting.

Teaching

Teaching and learning are the main work of all faculty and are a priority for all new educators (Scheetz, 2000). Many nurse educators teach theory and clinical and must develop teaching, learning, and evaluation methods for both areas. The teaching role is one that develops with time, experience, and knowledge and is in a constant state of growth and development. There are many factors that influence this process. Each teacher develops their own unique style that is influenced by personal beliefs, pedagogies, individual learner's styles, personal philosophy as well as the beliefs, pedagogies, and philosophy of their academic institution. Additionally, there is an ongoing commitment to identify new teaching pedagogies based on current research and technology. In an academic organization the faculty member is responsible for developing or revising course syllabi, selecting reading materials, developing course outlines, utilizing a variety of teaching strategies, professional role development, role modeling, and evaluation methods. Teaching effectiveness must also be demonstrated (Billings, 2008).

Teaching effectiveness is evaluated by student and peer evaluations, and student success. This will be further explored in Chapters 5 and 6.

Service

Service is a way of offering one's time or energy in the life of the college or the local, national, or global community. Service involves unpaid voluntary activities within or outside the college setting. Examples of service include serving on school of nursing committees or college-wide committees, mentoring new faculty, chairing a committee, serving on a board or advisory committee, serving on an international board, or speaking at local events (Billings, 2008). Although service is an important component of faculty promotion and tenure it is not weighed as heavily as teaching and scholarship. New faculty should volunteer for some activities but initially should focus on their development of excellence in their teaching role (see Chapter 14).

Scholarship

Scholarship is most often associated with research activities. Scholarship includes conducting research, obtaining grants, presentations of scholarly work, consultations, and published material (Billings, 2008). However, the AACN has a broader view of scholarship in academia. Based on the work of Boyer (1990) the AACN released a position paper in 1999 that addressed four areas of rigorous scholarly development standards for nurse faculty: scholarship of discovery, scholarship of teaching, scholarship of practice, and scholarship of integration (AACN, 1999). The scholarship of discovery involves research, inquiry, theory development, peer reviewed publications, mentoring, and grant awards. The scholarship of teaching involves knowledge of teaching learning theories, development of teaching and evaluation methods, program development, and role modeling. The scholarship of practice includes development of clinical knowledge, professional development, research skills, and service. The scholarship of integration includes interdisciplinary collaboration in discovery, practice, or teaching (AACN, 1999). As the nurse educator becomes a more experienced and proficient teacher he/she will be ready to make significant contributions to the advancement of nursing science (see Chapter 17).

MENTORS

Most successful people have had a mentor at some point in their life. "The original Mentor is a character in Homer's epic poem, *The Odyssey*. When Odysseus, King of Ithaca, went to fight in the Trojan War, he entrusted the care of his kingdom to Mentor. Mentor served as the teacher and overseer of Odysseus's son, Telemachus" (F. John Reh, About.com Guide, 2010, para. 4). A mentor can help the new nurse educator have a smoother transition into the academic setting. Mentoring is a reciprocal relationship that positively influences the development of self and career. For example, Vance and Olsen (1998) describe the mentoring relationship as the "gift-exchange phenomenon" (p. 3). The importance of mentoring and how to select a mentor will be discussed in greater detail in Chapter 15.

TIME MANAGEMENT

Time management can be quite challenging for full-time nurse educators. Even experienced nurse educators become overwhelmed at times. The big picture involves managing time spent on teaching, learning, and service. Planning for the semester is the next area to be organized. On a weekly basis formal teaching which includes preparation, presentation, and evaluation will equal approximately 40 hours. This amount of time will vary based on type of courses taught. For example, a theory course may involve 4 hours of face to face instruction every week whereas a clinical course may involve 12 hours of face to face instruction. Once the overall schedule is created the nurse educator has to plan out the weekly, daily, and course schedules. Added to this schedule is time spent at meetings, office hours, student advisement and mentoring, service, and scholarship. Strategies for organization and time management will be discussed further in Chapter 8.

ACADEMIC INTEGRITY

Academic integrity applies to institutions, faculty, and students. There are five values that must be embraced: honesty, trust, fairness, respect, and responsibility (Center for Academic Integrity [CAI], 1999, p. 4). Honesty applies to test taking, plagiarism, research, and misrepresentation. Trust must be established between faculty and students. Creating clear course guidelines and evaluation policies will help to build trust. Everyone must be treated fairly. Faculty must create concrete evaluation tools to grade students fairly. They must also address all violations of academic integrity. Creating a culture of mutual respect will foster a positive learning environment. All members of the academic community are responsible for creating and maintaining a culture of academic integrity. Breeches of academic integrity have been identified in colleges and universities across the country. Faculty must be aware of these issues and foster a positive learning environment where they create a culture of academic honesty through curriculum development and role modeling (Tippitt et al., 2009).

PROFESSIONAL ETHICS

Practically every profession has adopted a code of ethics in the past 20 years specific to their discipline. Rosenkoetter and Milsteid (2010) present a new code of ethics for nurse educators that was originally published in 1983. "The role of the nurse educator is to be a mentor, role model, information provider, and someone who challenges students to think critically about their ethical decisions and the ethical concerns of others whom they encounter in professional practice" (p. 2). The revised code has 17 standards and is an extension of the American Association *Code of ethics for nurses* and the *ICN code of ethics for nurses* (p. 2). Nurse educators can use the code of ethics as a guide in their pursuit of honesty, integrity, and ethical conduct in teaching, learning, and scholarly activities (see Chapter 11).

SUMMARY

Nurse educators teach in both academia and service. Each setting has a unique set of requirements and responsibilities. The academic setting is quite different from the service setting and many academic nurse educators begin their teaching role as hospital-based educators or adjunct clinical instructors. A master's degree is required in both settings with a doctoral degree as the terminal degree requirement for most academic settings. The three main areas that all nurse educators must excel in are teaching, service, and scholarship. In addition, nurse educators must be cognizant of tenure requirements, time management, academic integrity, and professional ethics.

DISCUSSION QUESTIONS

1. Compare and contrast the role of the nurse educator in both service and academe.
2. List five activities that would fall under the service category.
3. List five activities that would fall under the scholarship category.
4. Identify key issues in academic integrity.
5. Why is a mentor important?

SUGGESTED LEARNING ACTIVITIES

1. Review the Code of Ethics for Nurses—American Nurses Association. www. nursingworld.org/codeofethics
2. Review the ICN *Code of Ethics for Nurses.*
3. Review the *Code of Ethics for Nurse Educators.*
4. Read the 1940 *Statement of Principles on Academic Freedom and Tenure* at www.aaup.com.
5. Complete a self-assessment of your current teaching, service, and scholarship activities.

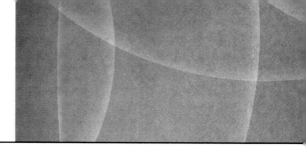

Personal Reflection of a Nurse Educator

VICKI MARTIN, MSN, RN

TRANSITIONING FROM A NURSING ROLE TO the nurse educator role can be very challenging. Upon entering academe, the nurse moves from a clinical-based nursing environment that requires patient-focused clinical management and care, to an educational arena that requires teaching, research, community service, scholarly activity, advisement, and participation in department/college committee meetings. This transition can be confusing, frustrating, and stressful for the novice nurse educator.

To be successful in the nurse educator role, it takes commitment to the university and to the students. Success requires good organizational skills and dedication to the curriculum. Every facility has a mentoring process, so new faculty should have a support person to assist with issues in a constructive and consultative manner. The mentor should be a seasoned faculty member willing to be a friend, coach, counselor, advisor, guide, director, teacher, exemplar, preceptor, and role model to the mentee for one year. A good relationship between the mentor and mentee is a crucial element for success during this phase of career building. The two should have weekly meetings to discuss the mentee's progress; to facilitate these meetings, it is helpful for both to have a similar or congruent teaching and clinical schedule. Without mentoring, this nurse educator might not have remained in academe.

Another element contributing to success for the new nurse educator is a desire to be a lifelong learner. This is necessary to remain current in practice, to provide evidence-based teaching in the classroom and clinical, and to provide students with an evidence-based foundation for competent and safe practice. Lifelong learning involves attending continuing education training and workshops, and a commitment to seeking more advanced degrees for personal/professional credentialing.

My best advice for new nurse educators is to be patient with yourself during the first year and realize that the learning curve will be steep. During this first year, you will learn to teach and discover that through teaching, you will also learn. Honing your organizational skills will help you to achieve balance between the quality and amount of work demanded in the classroom and with your students in the clinical settings.

The most important lessons I've learned in education are two: first, no one is going to die, unlike the clinical setting, and secondly, nurse educators are there for the students. Being a nurse educator is a rewarding, demanding, and time-consuming role. The experience of being a teacher is itself a great teacher. Teaching can be stimulating and gratifying, if you are willing to put forth the effort and time required to become an effective and seasoned academic faculty member.

REFERENCES

American Association of Colleges of Nursing. (1999). *Position statement on defining scholarship for the discipline of nursing.* Retrieved from http://www.AACN.com

American Association of Colleges of Nursing. (2010). *The nursing shortage.* Retrieved from http://www.AACN.com

American Association of University Professors. (2010). *Academic integrity.* Retrieved from http://www.aaup.com

Amos, L. (2005). American Association of Colleges of Nursing. *Baccalaureate nursing programs.* Retrieved from http://www.AACN.com

Bastable, S. (2003). Nurse as educator: Principles of teaching and learning for nursing practice. Sudbury, MA: Jones and Bartlett.

Billings, D. (2008). Developing your career as a nurse educator: The professional portfolio. *Journal of Continuing Education in Nursing, 39*(12), 532–533.

Boyer, E. (1990). Scholarship reconsidered: Priorities for the professoriate. Princeton, NJ: The Carnegie Foundation for the Advancement of Teaching.

Center for Academic Integrity. (1999). *Fundamental principles for academic integrity.* Retrieved from http://www.ethics.sandiego.edu/eac/Summer2000/Principles.htm

Gilbert, C. (2003). Nursing programs in America. *Medical Schools & Nursing Colleges Worldwide.* Retrieved from www.medical-colleges.net/nursing4.htm

Grad Schools.com 2010. Retrieved from www.gradschools.com/search-programs/nursing

Mahaffey, E. (2002). The relevance of associate degree nursing education: Past, present, future. *Online Journal of Issues in Nursing, 7*(2), Manuscript 2. Retrieved from www.nursingworld.org/ojin/MainMenuCategories/ANAMarketplace/

ANAPeriodicals/OJIN/TableofContents/Volume72002/No2May2002/RelevanceofAssociateDegree.aspx

McCloskey, J., & Grace, H. (1981). *Current issues in nursing.* Oxford: Blackwell Scientific Publications.

Neeb, K. (2006). *Mental health nursing* (3rd ed.). Philadelphia, PA: F.A. Davis Company.

Reh, J. (2012). Mentors and mentoring: What is a mentor? About.comManagement.

Rosenkoetter, M., & Milstead, J. (2010). A code of ethics for nurse educators: revised. *Nursing Ethics, 17*(1), 137–139. doi:10.1177/0969733009350946.

Scheetz, L. (2000). *Nursing faculty secrets.* Philadelphia, PA: Hanley & Belfus, Inc.

Siela, D., Keller, V., & Connolly, M. (2008). The shortage of nurses and nursing faculty: What critical care nurses do. *AACN Advanced Critical Care, 19*(1), 66–67.

Tippitt, M., Ard, N., Kline, J., Tilghman, J., Chamberlain, B., & Meagher, P. (2009). Creating environments that FOSTER academic integrity. *Nursing Education Perspectives, 30*(4), 239–244.

Vance, C., & Olsen, R. (1998). *The mentor connection in nursing.* New York, NY: Springer.

CHAPTER 2

Role Preparation

"Tell me and I forget. Teach me and I remember.
Involve me and I learn."

—BENJAMIN FRANKLIN

OBJECTIVES

After reading this chapter, the reader will be able to
- Discuss educational requirements for nurse faculty in academia
- Discuss educational requirements for nurse educators in non-academic settings
- Compare and contrast educational requirements for nurse educators in service and academia.
- Discuss how nursing experience relates to the teaching role
- Identify related educational experiences in the teaching role

INTRODUCTION

This chapter will focus on the specific educational requirements and experience that are required for nurse educator roles in both service and academia. Your current level of education and past experience will dictate where you will most likely begin your teaching career. Knowing the requirements will guide you in creating your short-term and long-term career goals. It is important to note that there are many different programs and one must be an educated consumer when choosing a program. You must select an accredited program so that it will be recognized as meeting the standards of academic rigor. Additional considerations in selecting a program include: location, philosophical beliefs of the program, financial support, and academic support services. This applies to all levels of education.

EDUCATIONAL REQUIREMENTS FOR HOSPITAL-BASED EDUCATORS

The educational requirement for hospital-based or non academic educators is most often a master's degree in nursing education. A master's degree in another related discipline may also be accepted with the caveat that the baccalaureate degree is in nursing. Completing a post master's certificate program in education is another way to meet the educational requirement for this role. The doctoral degree is often preferred, especially for nurse educator positions at the director level.

Some organizations will hire nurse educators who have a bachelor's degree and related experience with the expectation that the nurse educator will return to school for their advanced degree. In this situation the educator will be given a timeframe for completion and may or may not be eligible for tuition assistance. While this is a wonderful option for some, there is a certain amount of stress in continuing one's education while working in a new full-time position. Graduate studies are challenging and it can be overwhelming to attend school while working. Creating a plan with short- and long-term goals is very helpful. There are many factors involved in selecting a program of study and this will be discussed further at the end of the chapter.

EDUCATIONAL REQUIREMENTS FOR ACADEMIC NURSE EDUCATORS

The educational requirements for academia are more rigorous than for the hospital-based educator with the standard requirement being a master's degree with doctoral degree preferred.

The educational requirements vary based on the type of program. For example, in an associate degree or diploma program the terminal degree requirement is usually the master's degree although some institutions may allow baccalaureate prepared nurses to teach in adjunct roles. In baccalaureate degree programs, master's degree programs, and Doctoral Degree programs the terminal degree requirement is the doctoral degree for a full-time tenure track position. However, clinical instructors and adjunct faculty may teach in a baccalaureate program if they hold a master's degree in nursing with an education major being preferred (Penn, Wilson, & Rosseter, 2008). According to the American Association of Colleges of Nursing (AACN, 2008) nurse educators should have "graduate-level academic preparation and advanced expertise in the areas of content they teach." Because of the faculty shortage some academic settings will hire faculty who are clinical or content experts and are working towards a graduate degree. As a rule of thumb, educators should hold a degree at least one level higher than the program they are going to teach (Penn et al., 2008). However, if you are seriously considering a full-time tenure track faculty role, you should plan on obtaining your doctoral degree.

EDUCATIONAL REQUIREMENTS TO ACADEMIC EDUCATORS IN SPECIAL PROGRAMS

There are several special areas where nurse educators are needed to teach. For example, in a nurse practitioner program the nurse educators also need to be certified nurse practitioners. Therefore, the educational requirement would be the NP or DNP depending on the setting and Carnegie classification. Nurse practitioner programs have unique requirements and require an educator who is an experienced practitioner. The educator may serve as an adjunct or full-time faculty member.

Another area where adjuncts may be used is in a master's program for nursing leadership or administration. Often, highly experienced adjuncts that hold a master's degree in their specialty will be hired to teach one or two courses. In this case having a master's degree in nursing administration or a master's degree in business administration is highly desirable.

There are several areas, especially in an adjunct role, where a graduate degree in an area other than nursing education will be preferred. These include: holistic nursing, nursing informatics, clinical nurse specialist, palliative care, and geriatrics. In these highly specialized positions, academic settings seek experts to teach clinical and content.

NURSING EXPERIENCE AND TEACHING ROLE

Nursing is a unique profession and in this field nurse educators must have clinical experience before they may consider an educator role. The experience one has is invaluable and influences the future role of the nurse educator. In the current market, as healthcare and education are evolving the expectations are even greater. According to the National League for Nursing, "Tomorrow's nursing education must be research based, and it is best taught by individuals who are prepared for the faculty role and who demonstrate competence in the multiple components of that role" (NLN Position Paper, p. 195).

Nurse educators must complete their basic nursing education, pass the licensing exam, and work in service before considering a position in education. Furthermore, nurse educators should have at least two years of professional experience in their specialty area before they can consider a transition to education (Smith, 2005). Past clinical experience will dictate the type of courses the nurse educator will teach. For example, a nurse with experience in pediatrics would be hired to teach that content. A medical-surgical instructor would be required to have worked in a medical-surgical unit. Having certification in the area where one is hoping to teach will make you a stronger candidate.

QUALITIES OF A NURSE EDUCATOR

Nurse educators need to be well informed and stay current on all topics. It is a lifelong commitment and requires dedication and continued role development. A nurse educator needs to be knowledgeable about multiple teaching and learning pedagogies. Technology is playing a greater role in health care and education so nurse educators must develop the skills, knowledge, and attitudes to utilize technology in a variety of ways. Written and verbal communication are also a must for nurse educators. Being able to communicate with a diverse group of people is vital. This takes time and experience.

Scholarly writing must also be developed as publication will be expected and/ or required and nurse educators must help their students to develop their writing skills. Organization and time management are often the most challenging part but also two of the most important skills (Billings, 2008). There are multiple requirements and it is easy to become overwhelmed and fall behind. Investing in a planner and creating realistic objectives is the key to success. Being creative and flexible is another important quality for the nurse educator. Oftentimes, plans get changed, especially as a hospital-based educator and one must be prepared to adjust schedules and programs (NLN, 2005b).

ADVANCED DEGREES

There are many reasons to continue the academic journey, especially as a nurse educator. If being a nurse educator is your dream, then earning your doctoral degree should be included in your long-term goals. Recognizing the value and significance of increasing the number of nurses with advanced degrees, the Institute of Medicine (2010) published the Future of Nursing Report. This report was the result of collaboration between the Robert Wood Johnson Foundation and the Institute of Medicine. One of the four key areas identified was the advanced education of all nurses. Achieving higher levels of education will help nurses to play a more significant role in the development of policy and practice. The good news is that according to the AACN (2011) enrollment in doctoral programs has increased significantly in the past year.

HOW TO SELECT A GRADUATE PROGRAM

Once you decide that you want to return to school you need to begin searching the various schools and programs. Naturally, you will want to choose a school that is accredited, has a good reputation, and one that meets the needs of the adult learner. It is important to note that at least one of your degrees should be in nursing. So if you have a bachelor of arts degree, then you must complete your master's degree in nursing. Don't forget to find out whether the programs you are interested in will accept any previous credits. There is usually a timeframe of acceptance that ranges from 5-10 years. You may also be able to complete a challenge exam for some courses. Some other factors to consider are class and clinical schedules, library hours, the location of clinical sites, and parking (Hunt, 2006). You will need to create a master plan where you allocate time for work, family, and school obligations. If you goal is to become an academic educator, then you will need to earn your doctoral degree. However, if your goal is to have a dual role as a nurse practitioner and educator, then you may want to consider a DNP program. Next, you need to decide whether you are going to school on a part-time or full-time basis. Although you may want to go full-time to finish quickly, you don't want to set yourself up for failure. In most programs, you will need to achieve a grade of "C" or better to be eligible for tuition reimbursement and at least a 3.0 GPA to progress in the program, so you should give this some serious thought.

Part-time may turn out to be an attractive choice, especially if your employer offers tuition reimbursement. If you are considering a tuition assistance program, it's important to know that there is usually a cap on how much you may request in a semester or a year. Be sure to check out other financial options. There are some opportunities for scholarships but it is up to you to investigate with the financial aid office at your prospective educational organization.

Another fact to consider is the philosophy of the school and program of study at the school that you are considering. You may conduct an online search to elicit most of this information. It is important to evaluate if the philosophy and mission are in alignment with your expectations. If you are considering a research-based degree, then you will want to have an idea of a possible topic for your dissertation. You will also want to investigate if there are faculty members on staff who have similar research interests. It is most beneficial to have faculty who share similar research interests to guide and mentor you through this academic journey. You may also have an opportunity to serve as a research assistant with one of these faculties, which will provide you with an opportunity to learn more about your topic and the research process.

You may want to consider one of the many online courses; however, you need to confirm that the program is accredited and you must be disciplined enough to complete the work on your own. Many traditional programs have at least some offerings online. A thorough review of all programs should be done before making a final decision. Choosing the right school is critical; although you may be eager to start, it's time well spent when choosing the one that is best for you (Hunt, 2006). Developing a plan with short- and long-term goals will help you to identify your next preparatory steps. If you are completing your master's degree and wish to be an academic educator, you will seriously want to consider a doctoral program. If you are a nurse practitioner who wishes to teach in an academic setting, you might want to consider a DNP program. It is helpful to identify potential settings for employment so that you can discover which degree is accepted and or preferred. Keep in mind that many academic settings require that at least one of your degrees be in nursing. So if your bachelor's degree is not in nursing, you should attend a master's program with a focus in nursing.

SUMMARY

This chapter focused on role preparation. The specific requirements for different academic settings were discussed. An overview relating to nursing, clinical, and related educational experience was also presented.

DISCUSSION QUESTIONS

1. Discuss the various teaching roles and their requirements.
2. Discuss the relationship of clinical experience and teaching roles.
3. How might you select a nurse educator program?

4. Identify three of your strengths related to the nurse educator role.
5. Identify three areas for self-improvement.
6. Compare and contrast two different nurse educator roles.

SUGGESTED LEARNING ACTIVITIES

- Create a five-year plan for your role as a nurse educator with short- and long-term goals.
- Interview a faculty member from a college or university.
- Identify at least five potential academic programs that you would be interested in attending. These may be traditional or online courses.

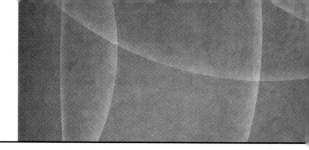

Transition From Practice to Education

CAROLE KENNER, PhD, RNC-NIC, FAAN

I CLEARLY REMEMBER THE TRANSITION FROM practice to education. I felt confident I knew the clinical skills and could teach in that setting, even undergraduates who always asked the why. But I was not confident I could teach in a classroom as I had no background for this type of teaching. Yet with a freshly minted masters degree I knew I wanted a foot in both camps: practice and education.

Today's new nurse educators face the same challenges I did. Yet with dwindling resources they may not be afforded the opportunities I had to team teach, and thus, to learn from experts. From them I also learned to "work smart." Every time I created new lecture material, I tried to envision an article or manuscript that could be published. I even co-wrote an article on my experience about moving from expert clinician to novice teacher. These activities helped me survive being hired into a tenure track position with only a master's degree with seven years to tenure and a doctorate.

Survive I did! Thrive I did! I had mentors to help me learn the faculty role, to guide me towards building my scholarship, and gain confidence in teaching. I had my students who kept encouraging me, and challenging me not to be afraid to admit I had no answers for some of their questions but I could find resources for them. Almost 30 years later I can honestly say I enjoy teaching. I miss the day to day action in clinical but I love seeing students learn. Now it is my role to mentor novice faculty in a rapid paced environment. I encourage new faculty to seek good mentors both internal and external to the organization in which they are employed.

I advise you to do the same: seek those who can offer you constructive criticism and help with a facet of your career. Seek opportunities to shadow fellow faculty, to gain from their expertise. If you are struggling in an area, seek help. Many times, we follow old adage: "see one, do one, teach one." Yet there are many of us who really want to help you on your journey but we do not know how unless you ask us. Remember too that if I am your supervisor I want you to succeed because it is a win-win for me, as well.

So trust in yourself, seek mentors, attend conferences to gain skills, and learn as much as you can and enjoy. You can touch so many lives through teaching because your students multiply your reach many times over in the lives of patients and families whom they touch. Teaching is like riding a roller coaster: enjoy the ride!

REFERENCES

American Association of Colleges of Nurses. (2011). New AACN Data Show an Enrollment Surge in Baccalaureate and Graduate Programs Amid Calls for More Highly Educated Nurses. Retrieved from www.aacn.nche.edu

American Association of Colleges of Nursing. (2008). *Position statement on the preferred vision of the professoriate in baccalaureate and graduate nursing programs.* Retrieved from www.aacn.nche.edu/Publications/positions/pre-ferredvision.htm

Billings, D. (2008). Developing your career as a nurse educator: The professional portfolio. *Journal of Continuing Education in Nursing, 39*(12), 532–533.

Hunt, D.A., (2006). The second time around. *Nursing Spectrum, 2*(14), 21.

Institute of Medicine (2010). The Future of Nursing Leading Change Advancing Health. Retrieved from www.iom.edu/nursing

National League for Nursing. (2005a). Transforming nursing education [Position statement]. *Nursing Education Perspectives, 26*(3), 195–197. [Online]. Retrieved from www.nln.org/aboutnln/PositionStatements/index.htm

National League for Nursing (NLN). (2005b). *Core competencies of nurse educators with tasks statements.* Retrieved from http://www.nln.org/profdev/corecom-petencies.pdf

Penn, B., Wilson, L., & Rosseter, R. (2008). Transitioning from nursing practice to a teaching role. *Online Journal of Issues in Nursing, 13*(3). Retrieved from CINAHL Plus with Full Text database

Smith, L. (2005). Joys of teaching nursing. *Nursing, 35*(134). Retrieved from MasterFILE Premier database.

CHAPTER 3

Testing the Waters

"Don't limit yourself. Many people limit themselves to what they think they can do. You can go as far as your mind lets you. What you believe, you can achieve."

—MARY KAY ASH

OBJECTIVES

After reading this chapter, the reader will be able to
- Identify educator roles in which to "test the waters"
- Discuss how to prepare for an interview for a teaching position
- Develop a patient education hand-out
- Discuss requirements and role of the adjunct clinical instructor

INTRODUCTION

This chapter will focus on types of ways to "test the waters" and to identify teaching roles for which you are best suited. Many nurses have a desire to become nurse educators but they are uncertain how and where to begin this journey or if they really have what it takes to become a nursing educator. Although some nurses may not realize it, all nurses are teachers in some respect.

In fact most nursing programs prepare their nursing students to be patient educators. This is an important role of the nurse and the foundational preparation for the role of nurse educator. Another informal teaching role many nurses participate in is the role of preceptor or mentor. Often there are formal preceptor programs offered to nurses who are interested in becoming preceptors. Even nurses who are not identified as formal preceptors will most likely spend some time assisting new nursing and ancillary staff during their orientation to the unit. Therefore, it is important to recognize the accessibility of assuming one or more of these roles to "test the waters." These roles include preceptor, patient educator, guest lecturer, and adjunct faculty.

PREPARATION AND EXPERIENCE

From the day you begin nursing school you are being prepared for a teaching role. In every clinical experience you will be expected to teach your patients about their health. This usually involves an assessment of the learner, teaching and demonstration, and evaluating whether the teaching has been effective. These are important developmental stages for all nurse educators. Many nursing students are also expected to participate in group projects where they teach their classmates about a particular topic. This is another invaluable

---

EXHIBIT 3.1

Self-Assessment of Skills and Competencies

Please check all that apply

__Clinical expertise in: _____

__Interpersonal skills

__Self-directed

__Knowledge of teaching and learning theories

__Knowledge of unique learning needs of the adult learner

__Knowledgeable about learning styles

__Excellent communication skills

__Past teaching experience in: _____

__Related educational experience: _____

__Excellent organization and time management skills

This checklist may be used as a self-assessment and to create a five-year plan.

Template Five-Year Career Plan (include educational and professional goals, measurable objectives, and a specific plan)

Long-Term Goals:	
Objective 1	
Objective 2	
Plan	
Short-Term Goals:	
Objective 1	
Objective 2	
Plan	

experience for nurses as it offers them an opportunity to teach in a formal setting. As nurses begin their professional careers, they continue to teach their patients, share knowledge with their peers, and play some role, either formally or informally, in the orientation of new staff members.

Collectively, all of your experience from nursing school to the time you decide to "test the waters," has prepared you for a nurse educator role. The type and duration of clinical experience contributes significantly to the direction the nurse educator journey will take. For example, if you are interested in becoming a clinical instructor in pediatrics, you will need to demonstrate nursing experience on a pediatric unit. This holds true for most adjunct positions, as positions in theory or clinical will require related experience for any individual to be considered for that position. Being certified in one's specialty is important in preparing for an educator position, in both clinical and classroom settings. It is helpful to complete a self-assessment of your skills and experiences prior to applying for any teaching role (see Exhibit 3.1).

TIME TO TEST THE WATERS

Once you have completed a self-assessment, it is time to consider what position you are qualified for at this point in time. It is important to consider the time commitments for whatever position you are interested in. For example, you may be interested in teaching a clinical course one day per week for an eight- or twelve-hour shift. However, you will need to consider the time spent on travel, preparation, and grading assignments and student performance. If you are interested in being a lecturer you will need more time to prepare lectures, create exams, grade papers, and evaluate student performance. The next step is to conduct a job search to locate possible opportunities. This may be done through a formal process or word of mouth. Jobs may be posted in nursing magazines and journals, and organizational websites. You can also sign up for notification through online services such as Careerbuilder.com. If you are interested in an adjunct position, then you should start with local colleges and universities that offer nursing programs. You will want to consider all options. The next step is to apply for the position with the submission of a cover letter and resume or curriculum vitae (see Chapter 4).

Development of a cover letter and resume/CV will be reviewed in further detail in the following chapter. Be sure to tailor each cover letter to the specific position you are applying for. You will want to check if the organization prefers to receive submissions via e-mail, facsimile, or regular mail. Many organizations have a total online application process, so be sure to use the preferred format.

TEACHING ROLES IN HEALTH CARE ORGANIZATIONS

Most hospitals have one or more nurse educators depending on the size of the organization. The nurse educator plays a pivotal role in the hospital setting and works closely with nursing administration. As previously discussed, the hospital-based educator is most often responsible for orientation, competency development, and continuing education. To be qualified for this type of role you need related experience and education. The requirements will vary based on the size and type of organization. Although a master's degree is preferred you may still be considered with a bachelor's degree, especially if you are enrolled in a program of study, preferably in a nurse educator track or a clinical nurse specialist. If you hold a master's degree that is not in education you may want to consider completing a post-master's certificate program in education.

Clinical experience is essential in obtaining your first teaching position in a healthcare organization. Having clinical expertise in one or more areas is invaluable. Obtaining certification in your specialty will also be viewed favorably. Take advantage of any and all opportunities to develop your teaching skills and build your resume. Becoming a preceptor is a great way to gain experience. There is usually a course offered and because of high turnover rates there are always new staff that need to be precepted. Join one or two hospital-wide committees, especially ones that relate to education. Volunteer to develop patient education materials (a template is located at the end of this chapter). Creating material for patient education is somewhat challenging as you have to find a balance between being overly complex and too simple. Perkins and Cohen (2008) investigated readability of written material used to teach nutrition to patients in a large teaching hospital. They concluded that "Simple, clear messages are most effective for all groups" (p. 219). Because education and literacy levels vary among patients most experts agree that teaching materials should be geared to a 6th–8th grade reading level and jargon should be avoided (Canobbio, 2006). Even when patients have advanced degrees and high reading levels they may not understand complex medical terms (DeMarco & Nystrom, 2010). Utilizing the SMOG formula for readability may be helpful in developing patient education material. The SMOG formula can be used to create patient education tools that are based on a person's level of education and comprehension. (Contreras, Garcia-Alonso, Echenique, & Daye-Contreras, 1999). Demir, Ozsaker, and Ilce (2008) conducted a study on patient education material for surgical patients. They found that a significant number of materials were deficient and in some clinics there were no materials available. They also posit that healthcare professionals should be the ones to develop patient education materials. Clearly, there is a need for well-developed patient education material.

Writing an article, especially a continuing education article for one of the nursing magazines or journals, is another option. Joining professional organizations that provide you with an opportunity to network, find mentors, and learn about job opportunities.

ALTERNATIVE TEACHING ROLES

There are many alternative teaching roles that one may consider. For example, there is always a need for CPR, BCLS, ACLS, and PALS instructors. The CPR and/or BCLS courses have the highest need so it is advisable to start there. There is often a requirement to be certified as a provider for one or two years prior to completing a course. Instructor courses are offered by many organizations and may be eligible for tuition reimbursement. In these courses you will learn various teaching pedagogies and principles of adult education. You will also have an opportunity to teach part of the course, and will have an opportunity to develop course objectives, teaching strategies, and evaluation methods. You may teach these courses for your organization, or become a freelance instructor.

Another possible teaching opportunity is to participate in health fairs, or volunteer to teach at local schools, libraries, and community centers. There are multiple topics one can teach about, especially in the community setting. Health promotion and wellness are a major focus of many community groups so this is an excellent time to get involved in these types of activities. Penn, Wilson, and Rosseter (2008) suggest volunteering in your organization's staff development department, or becoming a clinical preceptor for nursing students. Many schools utilize experienced nurses to be preceptors for senior nursing students during their capstone courses.

Many organizations focus on health care and education in other countries. Although these are most often short-term voluntary positions they are quite rewarding. These include but are not limited to Hope for a Healthier Humanity, Doctors Without Borders, Health Volunteers Overseas, and Action Against Hunger.

ADJUNCT CLINICAL INSTRUCTOR ROLE

If you have a desire to teach, do not be afraid. There will be plenty of mentors to help you along the way. Whether as an adjunct or full-time faculty member, you can make a difference and the rewards will far outweigh the sacrifices. Becoming a clinical instructor can be a wonderful way to test the waters. It's okay to be a novice. It gives you the opportunity to learn and grow. You are already an experienced nurse with a wealth of information and knowledge, and this experience will just broaden your horizons (Hunt, 2006). The clinical instructor role is a perfect place to start your academic teaching career. Nursing programs are always in need of highly experienced clinicians who can be responsible for the clinical experiences of the nursing students. Although teaching experience is still preferred, many colleges and universities will hire adjuncts who have a strong clinical background. Penn et al. (2008) recommend talking to other faculty members about potential places to teach. They also discuss the importance of exploring the school's rankings, accreditation, and faculty qualifications. It is important to select an organization that will offer some type of orientation and a good support system. For example, Cangelosi, Crocker, and Sorrell (2009) conducted a narrative inquiry study on 45 participants and concluded that novice nurse educators need support and mentoring in the transition to becoming expert teachers. Furthermore, being an expert clinician does not necessarily make someone an expert teacher.

The authors posit that "Education and mentoring are essential for nurses who are in the process of learning to teach" (p. 371). Janzen (2010) describes this process as one of transformation and uses the metaphor of "through the looking glass." She suggests that as one looks into the mirror one can see one's potential as a clinical educator. One can also look back on one's own experience as learners and think about the educators and mentors who taught one along the way. Kelly (2007) identifies nurse educator skills that focus on teaching, interpersonal, professional, and communication skills. Clinical nurse educators must be strong role models of good nursing skills and be capable of sharing their knowledge and expertise in the clinical setting. They play a vital role in the nursing program and the clinical development of the nursing program's students.

The following is a list of attributes that are required of all clinical instructors. New nurse faculty will continue to develop these skills as they gain experience in their new roles. However, it is important to have a basic proficiency in these areas as you begin your teaching role.

Attributes of the Clinical Instructor

- Clinical expertise
- Critical thinking and reasoning skills
- Strong interpersonal skills
- Excellent verbal and written skills
- Previous teaching experience
- Knowledge of teaching and learning theories of the adult learner
- Willingness to learn
- Understanding of learning styles
- Proficiency in technology
- Innovative and creative

The role of the clinical instructor may vary among organizations but the list below is representative of some of the responsibilities of the clinical instructor. It is important to understand your role and responsibilities and to be cognizant of the fact that there may be different requirements based on the organization.

Responsibilities of the Clinical Instructor

- Assignment planning
- Collaboration and communication with clinical site staff
- Following the policies and procedures of the clinical site
- Clinical instruction and guided learning experiences
- Facilitator
- Create a positive learning experience
- Maintain patient safety
- Student mentoring

- Student observation
- Being a role model
- Student evaluations
- Direct patient care with students
- Communicating student concerns to course coordinator
- Assessment and evaluation of student papers and learning outcomes

(Adapted from Hunt, Unpublished data; Penn et al., 2008)

DEVELOPING A PATIENT EDUCATION HAND-OUT

Patient education is something most nurses participate in and developing a patient education hand-out is a great experience for the aspiring educator. Often an interdisciplinary approach is advised. However, individual hand-outs can be developed and then submitted to a hospital-wide committee for comments and critique. Developing a patient education hand-out can be challenging because the material has to be written in such a way that it is neither too complex nor too simple. Many experts recommend writing to a fifth-grade level of comprehension and avoiding medical terms and jargon (Monsivais & Reynolds, 2003; Washburn, 2000).

Table 3.1 gives the characteristics of an ideal patient hand-out; it was developed by Perkins and Cohen (2008) and reprinted with permission from Jennifer Cohen, Oncology Dietitian, Department of Nutrition & Dietetics, Sydney Children's Hospital.

Table 3.1 Characteristics of the ideal educational resource

Characteristic	Qualities to incorporate
Content	• Present ideas logically, with one idea or issue in each paragraph • Messages should be simple, relevant, concise and easy to follow • Information should be accurate and up to date. Include publication date so that the resource can remain current
Readability level	• Aim for the resource to be between years 6 and 8 in reading level • Use the SMOG index to assess the resource • Peer review should be sought following development for further improvement
Words and phrases	• Use simple words and short sentences • Use every-day English and avoid medical jargon • Define medical terms • Avoid simplifying the text using expressions that may be simpler to read but are not common phrases • Use active voice and conversational tone

(continued)

Table 3.1 Characteristics of the ideal educational resource (*continued*)

Characteristic	Qualities to incorporate
Fonts	• Font size-14–16 for text and 16–18 for headings • Font type-Arial, Tahoma, Century Gothic, or Bookman Old Style
Layout	• Match content with headings • Allow ample space within text and between paragraphs • Use suitable pictures or tables that enhance understanding, support the educational message, and make it more visually pleasing
Paper	• Use dark print on a light background

Adapted with permission of Perkins and Cohen (2008, p. 216–221).

Exhibit 3.2 provides additional guidelines for developing patient education material and hand-outs.

EXHIBIT 3.2

Patient Education Tips

■ Use an active voice
■ Design an interesting cover. If the cover is not appealing, patients will not pick up the material.
■ Write chapter titles in the first person (e.g., "Why did I have a stroke?" or "Why is my body not working right?").
■ Use bullets or tables for information
■ Use as few words as possible to get messages across.
■ Be sure to use a large-sized type size (14 points) and black type for easier reading.
■ Include easy to understand pictures or charts

(Adapted from Stonecypher, 2009, p. 464)

SUMMARY

This chapter focused on ways to test the waters. There are many ways for a nurse to discover if becoming an educator is a role that he/she may find rewarding. There are many education-related roles that can be used to "test the waters," including becoming a preceptor, a mentor, an adjunct clinical instructor, and a patient educator.

DISCUSSION QUESTIONS

1. Discuss the various teaching roles in the hospital.
2. What are the key components of a patient teaching hand-out?
3. Discuss alternative teaching roles.
4. List five attributes of a clinical instructor.
5. List five responsibilities of a clinical educator.

SUGGESTED LEARNING ACTIVITIES

- Develop a patient education hand-out in the area of your expertise utilizing the guidelines in this chapter.
- Complete a self-assessment of your attributes.
- Identify at least two possible educator opportunities and develop an action plan on how to obtain this position.

Nursing Education

LAUNETTE WOOLFORDE, EdD(c), DNP, RN-BC

THE WORLD OF EDUCATION OFFERS A plethora of opportunities for nurses. Although we may default to thinking of education in its purist form—teaching in a classroom—education is inherent in nursing but the formal role or title of nurse educator can take on many shapes and forms. The ember of interest in nursing education can be ignited at any point in the career journey. For some it is what we always wanted to be, for others it's been a charge by another nurse leader who recognizes that educator talent. Still for others, the desire to become a nurse educator comes after years of practice, development of confidence and expertise, and a desire to share knowledge with others. Regardless of origin, a career is nursing education promises to be an enriching and rewarding experience.

I recognized my passion for nursing education when I began serving as a preceptor to nursing students while working as a staff nurse. Anytime there were students, I volunteered to work with them. I loved the energy of students, and I loved being able to share with them the wide variety of things that I was learning in my career journey. It brought me great satisfaction to see them learn and grow and to be a part of their "ah ha" moments! It was through this preceptor experience that I recognized that I loved nursing education. I continued my work as a preceptor but began to venture out into teaching roles in nursing. As I became more exposed and engaged in nursing education, I realized that education was both a skill and an art. The ability to impart information to others in a manner that holds their interest, that promotes retention of information, and more importantly, that supports their ability to apply the knowledge learned when situations arise, is a talent that (a) not everyone has, and (b) needs cultivation and development.

I knew that it would take more than being a good nurse to become a good nurse educator. I've often heard remarks such as "You really know your stuff. You should become an educator." And while that has its truths, becoming a good educator is just not that simple. As a nurse educator, you've got to figure out how you're going to transfer what you know so well to others so it becomes second nature to them. You've got to commit to lifelong learning, which means advancing your education academically and through continuing education, certification, participation in professional organizations, and more.

As a new nurse educator, you may ask yourself, "How am I supposed to know everything? How do I handle questions and situations when I'm not sure of the answer?"

I've learned that while nurse educators know a lot, they don't know everything. So becoming a good nurse educator involves knowing your resources and becoming a sound resource for information and problem solving. It's about finding the blend among education, research, and practice. Nurse educators are skilled in evidence-based practice and practice-based evidence. Nurse educators are recognized experts, so as a novice nurse educator you may wonder how you will make the leap from novice to expert. You will do so in small steps, and by utilizing success strategies such as mentorship and commitment. When I embarked on a career path in nursing education, I solidified my foundation with a degree in nursing education. I formalized my knowledge by studying nursing education on a post-master's and doctoral level. That's what nurse educators do! We embody and role model lifelong learning.

I was fortunate to find a wonderful mentor, someone I admired and wanted to emulate. But perhaps more importantly, my mentor recognized my talent and my commitment that she felt were worth nurturing. My mentor has played an integral role in my growth as a nurse educator, inspiring me to tell you: "Never underestimate the value of a mentor"! Finally, get a "whatever it takes" attitude. Grab opportunities to learn and grow, even if it is challenging. Get involved in everything you can handle professionally. These experiences will build a strong foundation that will prove to be priceless as you advance in your career journey in nursing education.

Nurse educators promote curiosity in learners and allow education to open the door for further inquiry. May you always have a strong desire for inquiry. First let that passion for inquiry serve as the impetus for your learning, then let it become the flame that you pass on to others through nursing education.

REFERENCES

Cangelosi, P. R., Crocker, S., & Sorrell, J. M. (2009). Expert to novice: Clinicians learning new roles as clinical nurse educators. *Nursing Education Perspectives,* *30*(6), 367–371. Retrieved from EBSCO*host*.

Canobbio, M. M. (2006). Mosby's Handbook of patient teaching. 3rd ed. St. Louis, MO: Mosby.

Contreras, A., Garcia-Alonso, R., Echenique, M., & Daye-Contreras, F. (1999). The SOL formulas for converting SMOG readability scores between health education materials written in Spanish, English, and French. *Journal of Health Communication, 4*(1), 21–29. doi:10.1080/108107399127066.

DeMarco, J., & Nystrom, M. (2010). The importance of health literacy in patient education. *Journal of Consumer Health on the Internet, 14*(3), 294–301. doi:10.1080/15398285.2010.502021.

Demir, F., Ozsaker, E., & Ilce, A. (2008). The quality and suitability of written educational materials for patients*. *Journal of Clinical Nursing, 17*(2), 259–265. doi:10.1111/j.1365-2702.2007.02044.x.

Hunt, D. A., (2006). The second time around. *Nursing Spectrum, 2*(14), 21.

Janzen, K. (2010). Alice through the looking glass: The influence of self and student understanding on role actualization among novice clinical nurse educators. *Journal of Continuing Education in Nursing, 41*(11), 517–523. doi:10.3928/00220124-20100701-07.

Kelly, S. P. (2007). The exemplary clinical instructor: A qualitative case study. *Journal of Physical Therapy Education, 21*(1), 63–69.

Monsivais, D., & Reynolds, A. (2003). Developing and evaluating patient education materials. *Journal of Continuing Education in Nursing, 34*(4), 172–176. Retrieved from EBSCO*host*.

Perkins, L., & Cohen, J. (2008). Meeting patient needs in the hospital setting- are written nutrition education resources too hard to understand? *Nutrition & Dietetics, 65*(3), 216–221. Retrieved from EBSCO*host*.

Penn, B., Wilson, L., & Rosseter, R., (2008). Transitioning from nursing practice to a teaching role. *OJIN: The Online Journal of Issues in Nursing, 13*(3), Manuscript 3. Retrieved from www.nursingworld.org/MainMenuCategories/ANAMarketplace/ANAPeriodicals/OJIN/TableofContents/vol132008/No3Sept08/NursingPracticetoNursingEducation.aspx.

Stonecypher, K. (2009). Creating a patient education tool. *Journal Of Continuing Education In Nursing, 40*(10), 462–467. doi:10.3928/00220124-20090923-06.

Washburn, P. V. (2000). How to improve patient education. *Hospital Topics, 78*(4), 5. Retrieved from EBSCO*host*.

ADDITIONAL READING

Patient Education Management (2008). Field testing, a must-do for on-target handouts. *Patient Education Management, 15*(12), 136–137. Retrieved from EBSCO*host*.

CHAPTER 4

The Interview Process

"Go confidently in the direction of your dreams.
Live the life you have imagined."

—HENRY DAVID THOREAU

OBJECTIVES

After reading this chapter, the reader will be able to:
- Discuss key components of the interview process
- Identify key differences between a resume and curriculum vitae
- Discuss key components of an interview
- Create a well developed resume/curriculum vitae
- Create a well developed cover letter

THE INTERVIEW PROCESS

The interview process for nurse educator positions varies based on the type of position being applied for and the type of institution offering the position. It is important to understand the variability of institutional hiring processes and the expectations of the individual organization. While health care and academic institutional expectations are somewhat similar, they differ in significant ways. Of course this depends on the type of position one is applying for within the organization. For example, the interview process for an adjunct teaching position is less complex than for a full-time faculty position.

APPLICATION PROCESS

The application process varies based on type of position and organization. Applications may be completed online, in person, or by mail. Some organizations have a specific online application and others prefer a cover letter and resume. In general, academic settings require a cover letter and curriculum vitae (CV), and non-academic settings require a cover letter and a resume. Applicants must conduct a search of all potential organizations to determine the requirements of the application process for each and then be sure to adhere to the required process. It is important to develop a well written resume or curriculum vitae and cover letter. The application should be addressed to the appropriate person or department.

Health Care Organizations

Many health care organizations have an online application process. A resume and cover letter are still required in addition to the online application. If there is no online option, the resume and cover letter may be faxed or mailed to the organization. The next step in the process will be an invitation to interview with the recruiter. A follow-up invitation may be extended for a second interview to be held with the manager, staff, and other key personnel. The interviews may be individual or in a group. You may also be asked to develop and present an educational offering for one of the interviews. You will be given guidelines and time to prepare for this but it is a good idea to think about what you might want to present if asked to do so.

Academic Settings

The major difference within the academic setting is that a curriculum vitae (CV) and cover letter are usually required. However, if the position being applied for is an adjunct position and the applicant is a new nurse educator who has no teaching experience, a resume may be acceptable. If the organization feels the applicant has potential, an invitation for an interview will be offered and the interview will be scheduled. For an adjunct position, the interview most often takes place with the clinical coordinator and then is followed by an interview with the dean, the assistant dean, or the department chair. If the position is for a full-time faculty appointment, the process is usually more formal and the initial interview will take place with the faculty search committee. Following a successful interview, the search committee will make a recommendation to the dean. The next interview then takes place with the dean, chairperson, or other decision-maker. Each candidate most likely will be asked to demonstrate teaching ability. This may be accomplished by teaching a small portion of a lecture on a topic related to your area of expertise. The audience may include faculty or faculty and students.

Tips to Preparing for a Demonstration Teaching Session:

- Prepare well for this demonstration.
- Inquire what level of technology use is appropriate to incorporate into your teaching demonstration.
- If basic technology such as PowerPoint is expected, prepare a course outline, write your PowerPoint presentation to support your content, and

allow time for plenty of practice prior to the demonstration date so you feel fully confident.
▧ This is your opportunity to demonstrate your abilities as a teacher, especially if you are a new educator.

The final interview may take place with a senior administrative team. The hiring process for academia is longer than for a clinical position, especially for a full-time position, and may take a few weeks.

RESUME DEVELOPMENT

A well developed and polished resume is the key to making a good first impression. Recruiters receive a plethora of resumes on a daily basis so it is important to takes steps to ensure that your resume stands out. You want to portray yourself in a positive way but it must be factual. Based on your resume, the recruiter will decide whether you should be called for an interview. Although there are different formats that you can choose for your resume, there are some qualities that are universally important. For example, the information must be accurate and current. Your resume should be free of spelling and grammatical errors and the paper should be of good quality (Ryan, 2011).

Shakoor (2001) states there are several types of resumes with chronological and functional being the most common.

▧ The chronological resume is typically preferred by most recruiters. In this type of resume, you list your experience and education in separate, but chronological order starting with the most recent experience first. The formatting is variable and many computer programs have templates to utilize (see end of chapter for sample).
▧ A functional resume demonstrates the applicant's skills or competencies. This type of resume is advisable when an applicant has significant experience. However, it may also be used by someone with limited experience or gaps in work experience to emphasize special skills.

When applying for a new nurse educator position, submitting a chronological resume is advised. The components of a chronological resume include the heading, objective, educational, and work experience. It is important to create a list of all related experience. You will also want to spend some time thinking about your roles and responsibilities at each position. Because the resume should be limited to one to two pages in length, it must be concise. Most often experience is listed in chronological order with the name of the organization and the position. Responsibilities are listed in bullet points and should begin with a verb. You may also include a list special skills, honors, activities, and certifications. If you have completed scholarly work, you should include that, as well. A sample is included at the end of this chapter, but it is a good idea to review several resumes prior to developing one. You should also have your mentor, or someone else who is knowledgeable, review your resume prior to submission. You may choose to list education or experience first. You may also wish to use a template or a consultant to help you create a very polished document.

CURRICULUM VITAE

The curriculum vitae (CV) is somewhat different than a resume and most often is used by academics, researchers, and medical professionals. It is considered a biographical summary of one's accomplishments as an educator and a scholar. A CV is much longer than a resume and includes areas of teaching, learning, and scholarship. A new educator may have a CV that is only a few pages long but a senior faculty member's CV may be quite lengthy (50 pages or longer). There is no standard format but there is certain information that should be included (see sample template at end of chapter). Major topics to include are education, awards, publication of scholarly work (include refereed/peer review and others), published books and chapters, presentations, grants, research, recent continuing education, certifications, and courses taught. Do not include personal information such as gender, age, or marital status (GRE Explorer, 2012).

COVER LETTERS

The cover letter is one of the most important documents you will create. Just think of the adage "first impressions mean a lot." Cover letters should always accompany a resume or CV The cover letter introduces you to the recruiter and highlights your accomplishments. It is a way for the recruiter to quickly discover your qualifications for the position. Because the cover letter is read before the resume or CV, it presents the first impression of you and your capabilities and helps the recruiter see your potential for the position. The cover letter demonstrates your level of interest and professionalism. If the recruiter likes the cover letter he/she will go on to review the resume/CV.

Your cover letter should meet some basic specifications:

- Address it to the recruiter or other appropriate person.
- Spell the addressee's name correctly and use the correct title.
- Restrict the length to approximately one page.
- Write in a professional manner.
- Tailor the content to the specific organization and position for which you are applying.
- Begin with an introduction of yourself and the position you are applying for.
- In the second paragraph, write your qualifications for the position.
- Print both your cover letter and resume/CV on good bond paper in white or ivory. Some experts advise ivory because it stands out in the pile of white papers. Also a heavier bond paper may be attractive to the recruiter as it demonstrates that you are serious about this position.

INTERVIEW STRATEGIES

There are a plethora of studies and articles that describe the interview process and strategies for success. The initial interview is extremely important and requires preparation and practice. Because all organizations are different, it is difficult to know exactly how the interview will proceed but there are some things that are universal. In a recent article on job chemistry four main areas were discussed. One might consider them the "4 Rs" of job interviews. The four "R's" are research, review, refresh, and reflect.

- The first "R" (*Research*) involves a search about the organization to increase one's knowledge about the nuances of the organization. This demonstrates that you are serious and interested in becoming a part of the company.
- The second "R" (*Review*) is related to your experience and how it is related to the position. You should be able to identify your strengths and weaknesses. You should also be able articulate why you are the right person for this position. Based on the research you performed on the company and the position, you should be prepared to demonstrate that you are the right candidate for this position.
- The third "R" (*Refresh*) relates to being able to discuss your past experiences in the work force. You will want to highlight significant accomplishments in your previous positions. For example, if you are a novice nurse educator you would want to highlight related experience such as clinical expertise, patient education, precepting, and any other related experience you have had in previous positions.
- The fourth "R" (*Reflect*) involves being prepared to demonstrate your interest in this job and why it appeals to you. It is important to prepare questions for the interview. This includes questions you would like to ask and questions you may have to answer. You will want to portray yourself in a positive light but be careful not to over-embellish your qualifications (p. 31 "More than chemistry," 2011).

SUMMARY

This chapter focussed on the interview process and reviewed the importance of preparing a resume and/or curriculum vitae, and cover letter. Strategies for a successful interview were also discussed.

DISCUSSION QUESTIONS

1. What is the difference between a resume and curriculum vitae?
2. When would you use a cover letter?
3. How might you prepare for an upcoming interview?
4. Identify three areas that you feel qualified to teach.

SUGGESTED LEARNING ACTIVITIES

- Create a five-year career plan.
- Develop a curriculum vitae.
- Update your current resume.
- Participate in a mock job interview. Students should apply for a fictional position and develop a cover letter and resume/CV. Mock interviews should be conducted with faculty member(s) and other classmates.

REFERENCES

GRE Explorer (2012). Curriculum Vitae: How to Write a CV. Retrieved from www. greexplorer.com/Curriculum-Vitae.html

Job interviews: more than just chemistry. (2011). *Chemistry in Australia, 78*(3), 30–31. Retrieved from EBSCOhost.

Ryan, B. (2011). Four ways to write a successful resume. *New Hampshire Business Review, 33*(4), 18. Retrieved from EBSCOhost.

Shakoor, T. (2001). Developing a professional resume and cover letter that work. *Black Collegian, 32*(1), 16. Retrieved from EBSCOhost.

ADDITIONAL READINGS

Bennett, J. B. (1992). The curriculum vitae. *College Teaching, 40*(4), 155.

Khoo, V. (2012). How to ... write winning cover letters and résumés. *Charter, 83*(5), 44–45.

APPENDICES

Sample Resume

Marybeth Stevens
1214 Sunset Trail
Somerset, NY 10987
654-987-4312
mstevens@olamail.com

OBJECTIVE:
Seeking a challenging position as a nurse educator in an academic setting.

CAREER PROFILE:
- Strong clinical background in Med-Surg and Critical Care.
- Excellent interpersonal and leadership skills.
- Strong analytical skills, capable of assessing conditions and implementing appropriate intervention.
- Resourceful problem solver capable of implementing solutions to complex problems.
- Excellent oral and written communication skills.

PROFESSIONAL EXPERIENCE:
General Hospital, Somerset, NJ
1996–Present
Staff Nurse

- Educate patients/families on health care needs, conditions, options etc.
- Provide assistance to Nursing Manager in the supervision of staff nurses.
- Provide patient care for 6–8 patients.
- Assisted in orientation of new staff members.
- Served as a preceptor to new nurses.
- Served as a member of the Patient Education Committee.

St. Marks Hospital, Spring Lake, NJ
1994–1998
Staff Nurse

- Provide patient care for 8–10 patients.
- Supervised ancillary personnel.
- Performed clinical tasks according to hospital policies.
- Assisted in the orientation of new staff members.
- Educate patients/families on health care needs, conditions, options etc.
- Served as a preceptor to new nurses.
- Assisted patients and family members in the education of health care needs.

EDUCATION:
Henderson College, Gatesville, NJ
1996–2006
Masters of Science in Nursing Education
New Jersey College, Silver Springs, NJ
1990–1994
Bachelor of Science in Nursing

CERTIFICATIONS
- BCLS instructor
- ACLS
- PALS
- Med-Surg

HONORS/AWARDS
- Best Preceptor Award (2008)—**General Hospital**

REFERENCES
Furnished upon request.

Curriculum Vitae (CV) Template

1. PERSONAL INFORMATION
  1.1 Name
  1.2 Social Security Number
  1.3 Mailing Address
  1.4 Employment
  1.5 Phone numbers and Internet address

2. LICENSURE

3. EDUCATION
  (please provide the year, degree, university/college, location for each degree)

4. MILITARY SERVICE RECORD

5. OTHER SPECIAL EDUCATIONAL EXPERIENCE
  (for example, a certification program completed; not continuing education hours)

6. ACADEMIC APPOINTMENTS OR OTHER SIGNIFICANT WORK EXPERIENCE
  (please start with the most recent; provide years of employment, title/position, name of employer, location)

7. COMPETITIVE GRANTS

8. REFEREED AND NON-REFEREED WORKS
  8.1 Books: Chapters in Books
  8.2 Books: Edited/Authored
  8.3 Journal Articles (refereed) International, National, Regional, State/Local (please categorize)
  8.4 Journal Articles (non-refereed)
  8.5 Published Abstracts
  8.6 Other (example: continuing education programs)
  8.7 Manuscripts in Preparation

9. CONFERENCE PAPERS (REFEREED WORKS)
  9.1 International (refereed)
  9.2 National and regional (refereed)
  9.3 State and local (refereed)

10. PRESENTATIONS (INVITED)

11. MEMBERSHIP: SCIENTIFIC, HONORARY, PROFESSIONAL SOCIETIES

12. SPECIAL AWARDS, FELLOWSHIPS, GRANTS, AND OTHER HONORS
(do not repeat competitive grants here)

13. COMMUNITY SERVICE

14. MAJOR COMMITTEES
   14.1 School/college
   14.2 University
   14.3 Professional

15. OTHER SIGNIFICANT SCHOLARLY, RESEARCH, OR ADMINIS-
TRATIVE EXPERIENCE

16. MAJOR TEACHING ASSIGNMENTS

17. REVIEW ACTIVITIES

18. CONSULTATIONS

19. CONTINUING EDUCATION
(please list most recent CE information for the last 2 years)

20. CLINICAL PRACTICE/PROFESSIONAL PRACTICE

Sample Cover Letter

Dr. Gloria Robinson

Search Committee Chairperson

Green University

2395 West Meadow Street

Madison, Wisconsin 43298

Dear Dr. Robinson,

I would like to apply for the full-time nursing instructor position that was advertised in *Higher Education* this week. I feel that this position is a good fit for me based on my education, experience, skills, and knowledge.

Although I have not taught formally in an academic setting, I have taught in a hospital setting. In my current role I am responsible for the assessment, implementation, and evaluation of educational programs for the development of staff, including in-service classes, orientation, continuing education, annual reviews, skills certification review courses, virtual learning, and staff development. I also hold a master's degree in nursing education and plan to return to school for my doctoral degree.

Thank you for considering this application and I look forward to meeting with you at your earliest convenience.

Sincerely,
Judith Gray

PART II

The Teaching Role

CHAPTER 5

Finding Your Niche

*"It is the supreme art of the teacher to awaken joy
in creative expression and knowledge."*

—ALBERT EINSTEIN

OBJECTIVES

After reading this chapter, the reader will be able to
- Identify ways to find your niche (Med-Surg, Community, Geriatrics)
- Understand the role of clinical educator
- Identify past experiences that all nurse educators utilize in the classroom
- Describe ways to teach a course with no prior experience in a topic

NEW BEGINNINGS

It is always helpful to begin teaching in your area of expertise, especially as a clinical instructor. This knowledge is the foundation upon which you will build. Once you are familiar with the content, you just have to develop your teaching strategies. You will also draw from your own experiences as a student. In fact, many nurse educators espouse the philosophy of the program where they earned their initial nursing degree and teach the way they were taught. Later, when they become more experienced, they develop their own philosophy and teaching style.

The role of clinical instructor is a great place to start because you are utilizing your clinical expertise and serving as a role model while sharing your knowledge and skills with the students. For most nurse educators this is a comfortable place to start. You can also bring with you enthusiasm and positive energy as you engage in the teaching-learning relationship with your students. Of course, there is more to it than just role modeling but you will develop those skills as you transition into your nurse educator role. Clinical instructors are usually assigned to teach in an area based on their clinical experience. Although curricula vary, the main theory and clinical courses in generic nursing programs include foundations (or fundamentals) of nursing, medical-surgical nursing, pediatric nursing, obstetrics or maternal-child nursing, psychiatric mental health nursing, nursing leadership, and community health nursing. Based on your experience, one of these areas will be the perfect discipline for you to begin your role as a clinical instructor. Clinical instructors work closely with the full-time faculty member and are assigned from 8–10 students per semester or rotation. The clinical instructor plays a very significant part in preparing nursing students for their future professional nursing roles. It can be very challenging and requires excellent organizational and time management skills. The instructor usually is responsible for setting clear expectations, creating assignments, observing and evaluating students' progress, ensuring patient safety, communicating with staff on unit, observing medication administration and other care, completing summative and formative student evaluations, and adhering to organizational policies and procedures.

Before beginning the clinical instructor assignment, the instructor must complete an orientation at the specific agency. This orientation varies depending on the agency (hospital or medical center), but usually involves at least a day or two of orientation. Teaching in an unfamiliar agency can be somewhat daunting at first. In addition to teaching students, the instructor needs to become familiar with the nuances of a new organization. It is a good idea to reach out to the nurse manager for guidance. The nurse manager/designee will share expectations with the instructor. The instructor will be responsible for adhering to these guidelines and for sharing them with the students. Sometimes instructors are adjuncts where they already work or have worked in the past. This can be quite helpful as they are already knowledgeable about the agency and its protocols, although it is important to remember that each unit is different, even within the same organization. The norm on one unit may be completely different from the norm on another unit.

CLINICAL INSTRUCTOR ROLE

The clinical rotation is the mainstay of all nursing schools. It is a rite of passage for nursing students. This experience usually is met with both enthusiasm and apprehension on the part of the student, and quite possibly, on the part of the instructor. Suddenly the student is like a fish out of water. One minute the student is in the "safe" cocoon of a simulated learning center with "Mrs. Chase." The next minute, they are with a living and breathing "Mrs. Chase" who happens to be ill and in need of competent nursing care. This can prove to be a daunting experience for the student. Incorporating certain strategies into the experience by the faculty can make a major difference for the students.

The clinical instructor plays a pivotal role throughout the whole experience. The instructor is like a director in a play and must know the expectations and philosophy of the program and follow the established set of clinical expectations and weekly objectives. Strategies to achieve this include:

- Align the clinical assignment in conjunction with the current theory being taught in the classroom and past experience of the student, whenever possible.
- Both the instructor and students must learn the policies and procedures of the facility.

- Form collegial relationships with the staff on the unit.
- Develop a checklist (see Exhibit 5.1) for each student to keep track of the student's individual practice and to assist with assignment planning.
- Allow time for assignment planning, individual student conferences and grading of papers.
- Strive to offer appropriate learning opportunities for all students. For example, the students may have recently learned about COPD and the instructor might assign a patient with that disease. Students may need to be observed performing suctioning or wound care.
- Divide clinical time amongst all students to ensure that each student has a similar learning experience. Therefore, the instructor must be realistic in creating the assignment and should develop a plan for how to accomplish this during the course of the semester.

EXHIBIT 5.1

Sample Checklist for Medical-Surgical Clinical

Skill	Dates Completed S U
Medication administration	
IV administration	
Care of the patient on a ventilator	
Suctioning (tracheal and oral)	
Care of the patient with a chest tube	
Care of the patient with a nasogastric tube	
Foley insertion	
Care of the patient on oxygen therapy	

(continued)

EXHIBIT 5.1

Sample Checklist for Medical-Surgical Clinical (continued)

Skill	Dates Completed S U
Vital signs	_____
ADLs	_____
Bed making	_____
Transfer and ambulation	_____
Dressing changes	_____
Patient assessment and health history	_____
Therapeutic communication	_____
Interpretation of data	_____
Assessment findings, lab values, and studies	_____
Nursing care plans	_____
Documentation	_____

_____

_____

Skill	Dates Completed S U
Patient education	_____

Skill	Dates Completed S U
Critical thinking	_____
Evidence-based practice	_____
Quality and safety	_____
Prioritization	_____
Organizational skills	_____
Time management	_____
Self development	_____
Leadership Skills	_____
Timely completion of required assignments	_____
Professional behavior	_____
Other	_____

_____

_____

_____

_____

_____

_____

_____

_____

The clinical instructor helps the student to apply theoretical knowledge and clinical skills in the delivery of safe and effective patient care. Although the role may vary based on the organization and the type of clinical experience, the role of the clinical instructor is somewhat similar across organizations. One inherent challenge of the clinical educator role is learning how to create a weekly patient assignment for the students. This may be done the night before or right before the start of the clinical day. The assignment should be clearly posted on the unit so that students and staff are aware of patient assignments and responsibilities (see sample assignment Exhibit 5.2). Clinical instructors must be knowledgeable about the overall curriculum and course level. The course syllabus may be utilized as a guide when completing the weekly patient assignments to help students to apply theoretical knowledge in the clinical setting. Ideally the students should be assigned patients that relate specifically to their theory course. The assignments should also vary in complexity and become more challenging throughout the semester. For example, in the medical-surgical rotation, weekly assignments should become more complex and offer the student a wide variety of experiences. Depending on the organization students may be observed by the clinical instructor or a registered nurse on the unit. In many clinical courses the students will be required to administer medications and they must be supervised by the instructor or a registered nurse. The instructor must decide how many he/she can safely observe for the day. Then he/she must keep track of who gave medications and ensure that each student meets the expectations of the rotation and give constant feedback and critique of performance. The clinical instructor guides the students in completing the assignment in a safe, organized, and timely manner. If the agency allows, the students may also be assigned to spend observational time in other units at the discretion of the instructor. These include, but are not limited to, the operating room, critical care units, cardiac catherization lab, and hemodialysis unit. Students should be challenged to become more independent each week. The student is usually assigned one patient in the beginning of the semester but this may be increased based on the level of the course and as the student becomes more competent and confident. Of course, this must be in agreement with school and clinical agency contractual agreements.

Clinical faculty usually are responsible for conducting pre- and post-conferences. Some nursing schools have specific guidelines for the clinical day. In pre-conference, an initial discussion occurs about the focus of the day and the patient assignment. The discussion may include a brief history, chief complaint, medical diagnosis path physiology, diagnostic and treatment protocols including medications, laboratory results, the client's response to their illness and treatment protocols, the client's priority problems that the student will assess that day, and a specified individualized plan of nursing care addressing the client's individualized needs. During the post-conference, the discussion focus is on the student's learning experiences in relation to their specific patient during that day's clinical. The discussion topics may include the client's response to

EXHIBIT 5.2

Sample Clinical Assignment

Date: _____ Shift: 7a–7p Unit: _____

Pre-Conference: _____ Post-Conference: _____

Student Name	Patient Initials	Diagnosis	Special Assignment
Jane Smith	L.O.	CHF	10 am meds/wound care
Rory Green	P.K.	Angina	12 pm meds/blood sugar QID
Lucy White	T.L	Pneumonia	10 am meds/ suctioning
Robert Falk	K.H	COPD	12 pm meds/chest pt
Peter Perry	M.S	Angina	2pm meds/rom
Grace Allen	J.N	Asthma	2pm meds/wound care
Patty Parker			Observation in OR/ PACU

the care they received as well as related topics that emerged during the clinical experience, such as legal, ethical, or political issues related to their patient care. Other topics may include student's responses to the experience with their clients, with classmates, the nursing staff, the health care delivery system, research findings and their use in the care of clients, and new technologies for diagnosing and treating disease. (See Exhibit 5.3 for an example of a typical 12 hour clinical day.)

Additional responsibilities of the clinical instructor include grading care plans and assignments, and completing formative and summative evaluations. Utilizing a grading rubric (see Exhibit 5.4 for example of a generic grading rubric) is highly recommended as it enables the faculty member to objectively evaluate the student's written work. A grading rubric is developed by the instructor specifically for the assignment. Although it takes time to develop a rubric, it is helpful for the students and the faculty because the expectations are very clear (Allen & Knight, 2009).

Issues with student performance must be addressed immediately and communicated to the course coordinator or other appropriate person. Most

EXHIBIT 5.3

Example of a 12-Hour Clinical Day

The following is a guide to in planning the 12-hour clinical day.

7:00 AM—Pre-Conference/Discuss patient assignments, focus for the day, patient safety, communication, special assignments, questions and answers

8:00 AM—Arrive on Unit /Get report from primary nurse

9:00 AM—Patient Assessment/Patient Care/ADL's/Treatments

10:00 AM—Medication Administration (assigned students)

11:00 AM—Documentation (if agency allows)

12:00 PM—Medication Administration (assigned students)

12:30 PM—Lunch

1:30 PM—Patient Care/Patient Education

3:00 PM—Chart Review, Care Plans/ ATI Review, Student Presentations

4:30 PM—Patient Care/Documentation

6:00 PM—Post-Conference/Discuss events of the day/ Meeting objectives of the day. Patients and Care Plans/Nursing Diagnosis/ Interviews/ Positive and Negative Reflections/ Student Accomplishments/Self-Evaluation and Instructor Feedback

EXHIBIT 5.4

Template for Grading Rubric

All scores should be justified with comments under the appropriate text box

	Excellent	Good	Needs Improvement	Unacceptable
Score	4	3	2	1
Content				

	Excellent	Good	Needs Improvement	Unacceptable
Introduction				
Main Topics				
Organization				
Spelling and Grammar				
APA				
References within 5 years				

This is a guide that would need to be tailored to your specific assignment!

schools *have very specific* policies and expectations for passing and failing a clinical course. Most clinical courses are pass/fail and the instructor must document any performance issues and communicate this to the appropriate person at their college or university. Anecdotal notes should also be kept throughout the semester. This enables the instructor to keep an accurate account and to see how the student has progressed over the semester. Anecdotal notes are also useful when completing the formative and summative evaluations of student performance. A form can be helpful in keeping track of student progress and assignments. (See Exhibit 5.5 for example of anecdotal notes.) All faculty are responsible for adhering to the policies set forth by the clinical site and the academic organization. Legal issues are discussed in Chapter 11. The role of the instructor can be challenging but can also be a rewarding and enriching experience.

EXHIBIT 5.5

Sample Anecdotal Form

Student Name: _____ Semester: _____

Attendance	1	2	3	4	5	6	7	8	9	10	11	12	13	14	15
Date	1/25	2/1													
Attended	Y	Y													

Pre-Conference: _____

Patient Assessment and Care: _____

Medication Administration Dates: _____

Procedures Dates: _____

Documentation: _____

Patient Education: _____

Interpersonal Communication: _____

Professionalism: _____

Post-Conference: _____

Observational Experiences: _____

Comments: _____

_____

_____

_____

Written Assignments:

Care Plans (5 due): ___1___ ___2___ ___3___ ___4___ ___5___

Journals (3 due): ___1___ ___2___ ___3___

Narrative Paper: _____

THE ROLE OF THE NURSING STUDENT

Clinical faculty help their students to understand their role while in the clinical setting and should clearly communicate student performance expectations. The nursing student under the guidance of the clinical faculty is responsible for his/her actions and for providing safe care to assigned patients. The student must now assimilate theory content and clinical skills and apply them into clinical practice. She/he must be prepared, focused, and committed to learn. Students must collaborate with the instructor, peers, and hospital personnel. The student must always conduct himself/herself in a professional manner. Being prepared will help the day go smoother. Typical items required are a stethoscope, watch, bandage scissors, a calculator, and comfortable shoes. A weekly assignment may include completion of a patient history, nursing assessment, and a Nursing Care Plan. The student must understand which tasks can be done independently and which ones need to be supervised by the instructor. For instance, a student nurse may never administer medications without the instructor, but after demonstrating competence may complete an assessment, including vital signs and basic care. The student should always check with the instructor to verify what tasks can be done independently and report any significant findings or changes in patient condition.

Although the instructor has the sole responsibility for the students, the staff nurses can impart a wealth of information on the students. The students and faculty need to develop good relationships with the staff. They will receive a patient report from the primary nurse and must keep them abreast of patient status. The primary nurse is still responsible for the patient and must know what tasks the student will be doing for the patient. Most nurses want to help the students because they have had similar experiences. However, there will be some hectic days when the staff is too busy for students. One must remember that they are guests of the unit and should not infringe on the staff's time and space. Students should feel comfortable asking questions and communicate learning needs to the instructor. It is also important to work collaboratively with the other students and the rest of the healthcare team. The typical healthcare team is like a big melting pot consisting of many different disciplines. Not only are their educational backgrounds different but so are their cultures and ethnic and religious backgrounds. Creating a clear set of expectations from the beginning of the clinical rotation will result in a positive learning experience for the faculty, students, and staff.

BUILDING BLOCKS FOR NURSE EDUCATORS

All of your past educational and clinical experiences are the building blocks for your role as a nurse educator. Formal education, both academic and role development, will guide you as you continue to develop your role. As you journey into the world of education you will tap into all of these past experiences. For example, past theoretical and clinical experiences will have a major impact on your own development as a nurse educator. Most often in the academic setting when teaching theory and clinical, nurse educators will teach content based on their past clinical experiences. Therefore, all faculty are most often selected to teach courses in their area of expertise. (Cangelosi, Crocker, & Sorrell, 2009). Of course, one must keep up to date with current research and teaching and learning theories but in regards to style, new educators will often emulate the teaching styles of their past mentors, role models, and teachers. However, as new nurse educators become more competent in their roles, they will develop a style that is unique and based on multiple factors. (Sheetz, 2000).

Nurse educators must also continue to develop their expertise in verbal, non-verbal, and written communication. Most educational settings are diverse and nurse educators must be able to clearly articulate and develop course syllabi, lesson plans, and lectures in addition to writing reports and grading student's papers. In the academic setting many schools have templates to use as a guide for developing course syllabi which may be written individually or in collaboration with other faculty. In clinical courses the syllabus is most often developed by the course coordinator or faculty who is responsible for teaching the theoretical component. It is important to note that the course syllabus is a contract between faculty and students and must be strictly followed. Nurse educators must also be able to create methods for testing and evaluation. (Billings, 2008).

Nurse educators will continue to build and develop their roles as teachers by building on all of their past teaching experiences. These experiences may include patient/family teaching, mentoring, and presentations. Patient teaching is something many nurses do on a daily basis and new nurse educators have knowledge of the theories of the adult learner and will continue to develop based on this foundational experience. (Sheetz, 2000; Vance & Olson, 1998).

TEACHING NEW CONTENT

There are times when nurse educators in both the academic and non-academic setting will be required to teach a course or content in which they have limited expertise. This may seem daunting but it can be done, especially in today's age of information. When faced with teaching new or unfamiliar content, nurse educators will need to spend time researching and reading about the topic. Another faculty member or expert in the particular field may also be a great resource for learning about a new topic and for sharing course outlines, syllabi, teaching and learning strategies, and assessment tools. Auditing a course in a similar topic prior to teaching it may also be helpful. In adult education the faculty role is often one of facilitator so although you may not be an expert in the topic you will be able to develop a course and guide learning through the various teaching and evaluation methods and assignments. A rich classroom is one is which teaching and learning is reciprocal between the educator and the learners. Guest speakers are also a good option for content that is particularly challenging. Today most textbooks have a great wealth of information and supplemental materials available to nurse educators. Often times there are guides on how to teach the course, teaching strategies, key points, and even PowerPoint slides that can be tailored to your specific course objectives. Joining a professional organization may also be helpful as there will be resources and experts that may be able to offer guidance in the development of a new course. It is always challenging to teach something for the first time but there are many resources you can utilize and each time you teach the course you will become more comfortable and proficient with the content.

SUMMARY

This chapter focused on finding one's niche based on clinical expertise and presented an overview of the clinical nurse educator role. It also reviewed foundational requirements for all nurse educators and strategies to teaching unfamiliar content.

DISCUSSION QUESTIONS

1. Discuss ways to find your niche as a new educator.
2. Describe the role of the clinical nurse educator.
3. List at least five responsibilities of the clinical nurse educator.
4. Discuss key attributes of all nurse educators.
5. Describe three ways to prepare for a new course.

SUGGESTED LEARNING ACTIVITIES

▪ Develop a list of your areas of expertise.
▪ Develop a grading rubric using the template design (see Exhibit 5.4).

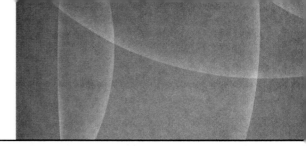

Reflections About Scholarship, Teaching, and Service: The Expectations of Academic Nursing

DEBORAH WITT SHERMAN, PhD, CRNP, ANP-BC, ACHPN, FAAN

IT WAS THROUGH QUIET REFLECTION IN a qualitative research class that I realized why I am a nursing educator. From the time I was a young girl, I imagined myself as a teacher. At that time, the majority of women who sought a career were advised to be a teacher or nurse. The only role models I had were women who were nuns or lay women teaching in the Catholic schools I attended. I "played" school constantly: making lesson plans, asking imaginary students questions, grading papers of my friends who played with me, or decorating the bulletin boards in my basement.

At age 11, a bicycle accident nearly took my life. It was the nurses, with their crisp white uniforms, white stockings and shoes, wearing a wide variety of interesting nursing caps, who would change my dressings, catheterize me, medicate me for pain, and comfort my fears. Three months after admission to the ICU and a subsequent transfer to the pediatric unit, I took my first steps toward becoming a nurse: I played with the babies of the unit, notified the nurse of a problem with another child, and offered comfort and encouragement to other children my age. Indeed, my nursing of others was so recognized that on the day of discharge, the nurses of the unit gave me my own nurse's cap. From that day forward, my life plan was that I was to become a nurse—and so it was to be.

During this personal reflection of my life, I had the first conscious realization of how I really became a nurse educator. By age 15, I was introduced to a woman who was a nursing professor. This introduction planted the idea of combining nursing and education. I would become a nurse and eventually would teach others the science and art of nursing. In completing my bachelor's degree in nursing, I taught my first class of a group nurses at a community hospital regarding death and dying, followed by a class to young parents about the care of their babies. Following the birth my first child, my passion for motherhood, nursing, and teaching led to my certification as a Lamaze childbirth educator. The nurse-educator story continued as I became a clinical instructor, later received a doctoral degree in nursing, and over time was promoted from an assistant to an associate professor and ultimately to a full professor.

The importance of sharing this story is that I believe reflecting on life's journey is very important. It is only by reflecting on the past, that we come to understand the present and envision the future. It is a building on life experiences, educational opportunities and experiences, and by challenging ourselves that we create our future, imagining the best we can be. During my first interview for a faculty position following the completion of my PhD, the Dean asked, "Where do you see yourself at the end of your career?" and I responded "I am going to be a dean," and she smiled. We must constantly envision the possibilities, create our reality, and reach for the "golden ring"—striving to grow and actualize our potential as men and women of nursing.

My passion is nursing—the comprehensive, holistic care of all people, everywhere, as I learned from the nursing theorist, Martha Rogers. To be the very best, I had to learn all that I could. Receiving a PhD in nursing was the highest degree that I could achieve in the profession. As doctoral students, we were expected to conduct a research study, but doing research was not my only focus or interest. As an assistant professor on a tenured-track line, I realized that developing a successful program of research was the primary expectation of academia that would lead to promotion and tenure. Yet, practice, teaching, and research were integral to each other involving an understanding of human phenomena of interest to nursing through clinical practice, educating nursing students as they synthesized knowledge from the sciences and humanities to provide excellent care, and generating new knowledge and translating that knowledge through evidence-based practice—indeed, the trinity of practice, teaching, and research.

Universities and colleges have a tripartite expectation of the scholarship, teaching, and service of faculty. In the first few years as an assistant professor, either on a clinical or research track, you understand the importance of advancing your scholarship.

- On a research track, your scholarship involves the funding of grant proposals in your area of specialization. Your publications will be data-based as you report on the results of your study and the implications for practice or further research.

■ On a clinical track, your scholarship may involve conducting quality improvement initiatives or collaborating with research faculty to identify important clinical problems and assist in the design or implementation of a study. The publications of clinical faculty will inform clinical practice, as you address the care of a particular patient population or focus on a particular clinical issue.

■ Both research and clinical faculty further disseminate knowledge through local, regional, national, or international presentations. Achieving the milestones related to scholarship creates significant anxiety for faculty—securing funding—getting published—and being invited to present your work. This is a challenge that is not for the faint of heart, as it requires motivation, persistence, and the ability to handle rejection without losing the spirit needed to submit, revise, and resubmit. It is important to understand that critique and feedback of your work are well-intentioned by reviewers and not a personal assault. Your resilience is central to your ultimate success in terms of scholarship.

Teaching is central to the mission of educational institutions. Teaching is more than the "transfer of information from the notebook of the faculty, to the notebook of the student without passing through the minds of either." It is the transfer of an appreciation for critical reading, critical thinking, and all that both processes involve: openness, honesty, appraisal, acceptance of varying perspectives, fairness, being non-judgmental, as well as recognizing the hazards of premature conclusions and closures. Teaching is reaching into the minds and hearts of students, captivating them with stories, helping them to get in touch with their intuitive selves, and creating the best conditions for learning with respect for varying learning styles, goals, and aspirations. Teaching is bringing out the best in a person, and helping them to see their potential, while guiding, and showing them the way through your own example—role modeling the values, attitudes, and behaviors of humanism, professionalism, and excellence in nursing. Clinical teaching, classroom teaching, or online classes are very different contexts, each with their own challenges and opportunities for the wonderful exchange between faculty and students. What I have come to realize is that experiential learning, and articulating ideas in writing or the spoken word, are the strongest ways of imprinting the mind and heart with the knowledge, attitudes, and skills necessary for excellence as nurses. As faculty, each semester provides opportunities to critically appraise your own knowledge, skills, and success in reaching your students and helping them to advance from novices to experts. Like your students, who are learning to be nurses, faculty are constantly in a process of becoming as their knowledge also deepens, and they gain an understanding of the most successful ways of sharing their passion for nursing and promoting their students' success.

In the beginning years as new faculty, clearly the focus is on scholarship and teaching. You have to excel in these areas if you are to be promoted or tenured. Yet, there are competing expectations of advising students, serving on school, university, or community committees, as well as participation in professional organizations. To achieve the mission of academic institutions requires the intellectual muscle and energies of faculty to ensure quality educational outcomes and the creation of a supportive, innovative, learning community. Department chairs need to protect the time of new faculty who must prove themselves in terms of scholarship and teaching. Learning to say "no" or other phrases such as "I would love to help at a later time—a year or two from now"—are not easy for new faculty who want to be good citizens and team players, yet feel excessive pressures for excellence in scholarship and teaching. Although service is valued and necessary, it is important for junior faculty or new faculty to be mentored regarding the areas of service that will establish collaborative networks. By strategic planning of service activities, faculty can be seen as contributors to the academic and other communities, but in ways that are consistent with their scholarly endeavors and which will enhance their teaching competency.

In conclusion, begin by understanding yourself, your path, how you got to where you are and how to reach your destination in terms of career goals and aspirations. Understand the importance of scholarship to the discovery of new knowledge and the integration of knowledge into comprehensive, quality care. The old saying "see one, do one, teach one" takes on new meaning as seeing, doing, teaching is influenced by the technology of our modern world and the realization that there are many ways of knowing according to Carper— empirical, aesthetic, ethical, and personal knowledge. As nurse educators, you are the facilitators of many ways of knowing—your own learning and teaching is constantly informed by the feedback of appraisal by your students and colleagues—both faculty and students mutually learning and advancing to experts in nursing. Teaching connects the minds and hearts of all who participate. Service is a process of involvement and engagement with the offering of intellectual insights, heart-felt concern for achieving the very best, and being responsible and accountable for developing the products or outcomes needed to ensure the vitality and vibrancy of a truly innovative learning community. Being selective in service enables faculty to integrate scholarship, teaching, and service while achieving the right balance that fulfills the goals of the individual and meets or exceeds the expectations of academia. Being new faculty is like learning a dance—eventually the awkwardness passes, you get in step with your academic partner, and your movements become graceful and fluid as your energy and spirits are synchronized—you wonder how you achieved this level of comfort and expertise—it is a complex process of synthesis that time allows to happen—enjoy every step, every move—with your partners sharing academic life.

REFERENCES

Allen, S., & Knight, J. (2009). A method for collaboratively developing and validating a rubric. *International Journal for the Scholarship of Teaching & Learning, 3*(2), 1–17, p. 56.

Billings, D. (2008). Developing your career as a nurse educator. The professional Portfolio. *Journal of Continuing Education in Nursing,* 39(12), 532–533.

Cangelosi, P. R., Crocker, S., & Sorrell, J. M. (2009). Expert to novice: Clinicians learning new roles as clinical nurse educators. *Nursing Education Perspectives, 30*(6), 367–371.

Scheetz, L., (2000). *Nursing faculty secrets.* Philadelphia, PA: Hanley & Belfus.

Vance, C., & Olsen, R. (1998). *The mentor connection in nursing.* New York: Springer.

ADDITIONAL READING

Foret Giddens, J., & Lobo, M. (2008). Analyzing graduate student trends in written paper evaluation. *Journal of Nursing Education, 47*(10), 480–483.

CHAPTER 6

Teaching and Learning Theories

"By learning you will teach, by teaching you will learn."

—LATIN PROVERB

OBJECTIVES

After reading this chapter the reader will be able to
- Discuss the following paradigms: behaviorism, cognitive, constructivism, humanistic theory, critical social theory
- Discuss Malcolm Knowles' principles of the adult learner
- Discuss teaching strategies for the adult learner

INTRODUCTION

There is a wealth of literature that addresses philosophies and theories in teaching and learning. If you consider an umbrella, you might picture philosophical beliefs (world view) at the top and underneath this umbrella are the various principles and theories of the adult learner. Most often educators utilize a variety of teaching and learning theories to best meet the needs of a diverse student body. Educational philosophies are sometimes abstract but they are the underpinning for the various teaching and learning theories. Possessing a basic understanding of these philosophical beliefs will serve as a guide in your own role development as an educator. A brief overview of philosophies and theories will be presented in this chapter.

PARADIGMS

A paradigm is as a worldview and can be used to describe the framework of a discipline. For example, Shuttleworth (2008) describes it in the following way, "A scientific paradigm, in the most basic sense of the word, is a framework containing all of the commonly accepted views about a subject, a structure of what direction research should take and how it should be performed" (p. 1). The paradigm of nursing includes: individual, care, environment, and nurse.

This paradigm refers to the professional practice of nursing and as such influences nursing education. Paradigms in nursing education have continued to evolve in response to advances in technology, medicine, and nursing science. Nursing education is in the midst of a paradigm shift. For example, Stanley and Dougherty (2010) posit "educators are rethinking historically teacher-centered curricular designs and are embracing new ideologies that have a stronger focus on student centered learning" (p. 378). However, it is important to note that because of the diverse backgrounds of nurse educators and students that span the generations, there are different educational paradigms and theories embraced by nurse educators. These are influenced by the nurse educators' past learning experiences, worldviews, and philosophical beliefs of the programs where one is a student or teacher.

Teaching and learning theories are developed under the umbrella of a philosophical belief. An overview of some of the well known beliefs will be presented within this chapter.

This will enable the reader to understand the differences and influences of these philosophies in nursing education. Although the philosophical beliefs are somewhat abstract they do influence your beliefs and practices as an educator.

EDUCATIONAL PHILOSOPHY

From the days of Aristotle philosophical beliefs have guided the development of educational theories. There are three main areas of philosophy: metaphysics, which is the study of the nature of reality; epistemology, which is the study of the nature of knowledge; and axiology, which is the study of the nature of values. The two main philosophical beliefs that have been embraced by nurse educators and have guided theoretical frameworks and pedagogies are idealism and realism (Melies, 2007). "Idealism states that the individual has a desire to live in a perfect world of high ideals, beauty, and art. Idealism focuses on truth as universal" (Billings & Halstead, 2009, p. 109). Realism has its roots in the educational and philosophical beliefs in the teachings of Aristotle. In realism there is a quest for knowledge and beliefs are based on scientific inquiry and the use of scientific method. Teachers who subscribe to the realist philosophy are very organized and concrete thinkers. Conversely, idealism focuses on existence of knowledge and the development of the mind. Idealists focus on truth and beliefs and understanding the world and tend to think more abstractly. Eucken and Phelps (1880) discussed the differences between idealism and realism. In idealism, knowledge and/or ideas are part of the phenomena that exist in our own reality. Realism is the belief that the phenomenal world exists independently of our minds. For example, an object such as a tree exists even if we do not know in our minds what a tree is (Smith, 2009).

ESSENTIALISM

Essentialism is rooted in both idealism and realism and considers both the mind and body as important foci in education. Furthermore, individuals are instilled with core knowledge and the view is that a student's mind may be molded or stretched to accommodate the information that is given by their teachers. In this approach the teacher is charged with imparting knowledge to the students. The student is like a sponge that must absorb the information that is given by the teacher. Preservation of core skills and knowledge is important and teachers give the students the essential moral and academic knowledge needed to fulfill their roles in society (Uys & Gwele, 2005).

BEHAVIORISM

Behaviorism is a theoretical framework that has its basis in realism. It has been a driving force in nursing education for the past 50 years. In this theory knowledge acquisition must be observable and measurable and is achieved through memorization and recitation. The roles of teacher and student are clearly defined with the faculty member guiding the entire experience. Furthermore, the approach is systematic and has clearly stated goals and objectives and learning takes place in a highly organized fashion (Driscoll, 2000; Eddy, 2002). Education focuses on motivating and conditioning the student to learn and the student is somewhat passive. In this approach the central role is placed on the teacher and the student is like a sponge that absorbs knowledge. When students do well they are rewarded for their behavior to reinforce learning. Tabak, Adi, and Edenfield (2003) posit that nurse educators have clung to the positivist views unlike the disciplines of sociology and philosophy, which have shifted to a postmodernist view of education that includes the scientific method or the human potential movement.

MORAL AND SOCIAL LEARNING THEORIES

Theories that address ethical issues are also utilized by nurse educators. Kohlberg's theory of moral development and Bandura's theory of social learning are two such theories that have influenced the moral and ethical education of nurses. Kohlberg's Theory of Moral Development addresses the development of morals from adolescence through adulthood. Nurse educators must consider the moral and ethical development of their students. Kohlberg's theory involves six stages of moral development that were based on Piaget's stages of moral judgment.

The six stages include: obedience and punishment orientation; individualism and exchange; cognitive good interpersonal relationships; maintaining the social order; social contract and individual rights; and universal principles. The learner develops and achieves these stages as they advance through their academic development (Bastable, 2003; Kretchmar, 2008).

Bandura's theory of social learning blended behaviorism and cognitive theories. In this theory the four components of observational learning are attention, retention, motor reproduction, and motivation/reproduction (Kretchmar, 2008).

CRITICAL SOCIAL THEORY

Critical social theory has been used to guide nursing education. Mooney and Nolan (2006) discussed critical social theory in nursing education. Traditionally nurses have been viewed as an oppressed group in relation to occupation, class, and gender. Furthermore, nursing education has perpetuated this oppression by the very nature of adhering to past traditions of teaching nursing. Freire's goal was to empower students and help students to be autonomous. According to Freire, praxis was the key to liberation. Critical praxis involves synchronized reflection and action. This provides a basis for how one comes to know and guides one toward liberation. Oppression in nursing has been fostered by the use of the biomedical model and educators who continued to use traditional approaches to education. Oppression can lead to aggression and complaint that is directed within the group instead of at the oppressors. "Freire (1972) noted that the education process could act as a tool for conformity or an instrument for liberation and promoted an education based on liberation, whereby individuals are empowered through critical examination of their reality" (as cited in Mooney & Nolan, 2006, p. 241). The role of the educator is key to this process. The educator must be reflective and communicative to foster students' growth and enable students to think critically and become independent in their thoughts. The educators must also become empowered so that they can enable their students to become empowered. Developing educational programs that have been influenced by Freire can help nursing achieve this goal. Professional growth and development can be realized through the use of critical social theory. Nurses must continue to grow and further define their body of knowledge in order to overcome prejudices that have existed in the past. Emancipation and knowledge development can be achieved with critical engagement. In 2002, Ireland moved to an all graduate nursing profession. This was consistent with trends in other countries that were concerned with the current education and the need for creative approaches to be undertaken in the education of nurses (Mooney & Nolan, 2006). A key component to nursing education is the liberation of students and the shift away from traditional oppressive education models. Nurse scientists through the lens of critical social theory have realized the significance of this finding. Nursing education is at a crossroads and continued efforts must be made to empower educators to adapt new methods for collaborating with students and thereby foster autonomy. The use of critical social theory is one way of achieving this goal of advancing nursing science and creating new approaches to nursing education (Mooney & Nolan, 2006).

HUMANISTIC LEARNING THEORY

Humanistic theory is based on the philosophical belief that all individuals want to learn and develop in a positive way (Bastable, 2003). In humanistic learning theory education is focused on empowering the students to be self-directed and have the ability to be autonomous in their decision-making.

The focus is on the student's personal growth and learning and enables the student to be self-motivated and creative (DiCarvallo, 1991; Li, 2007). The hierarchy of needs identified by Maslow influenced the development of humanistic learning theory (Milheim, 2011). The teacher's role is more of facilitator and is based on the assumption that students are motivated to learn. Humanism is the basis of many online classrooms in which the role of the teacher is that of a facilitator. But it is also applicable in traditional classroom settings, especially with the adult learner.

CONSTRUCTIVISM

Constructivism is based on the work of Piaget and has influenced the development of cognitive theories and adult learning theories (Brandon & All, 2010). "The major theme is that learning should be an active process in which learners construct new ideas or concepts based upon their current or past knowledge" (p. 90). The constructivist point of view is that the faculty member should function more as a facilitator and that the student should be an active learner. Furthermore, there should be a rich exchange between faculty and students that is based on problem solving and constructing of knowledge. Nurse educators might use concept mapping or case studies to help students to construct their own knowledge and to become active participants in their own development. Brandon and All (2010) discuss the constructivist model as a spiral in which the student is at the center and the educator creates meaningful experiences for the student to develop and eventually become expert learners. There are four guiding assumptions: student learning is based upon their past experiences; new constructs are formed through assimilation; students learn or construct knowledge instead of memorizing; and lastly, learning takes place through reflection and developing new knowledge that builds upon previously learned concepts. Furthermore, this type of learning helps students to develop critical thinking skills. Utilizing a constructivist approach can help nurse educators to shift from a content-laden curriculum to one that is student-centered and conceptual and fosters active learning, and critical thinking. This type of approach works well with adult learners who value autonomy and collaboration in learning.

ANDRAGOGY, MALCOLM KNOWLES, AND THE ADULT LEARNER

The theory of andragogy is based on the unique needs of the adult learner. "Malcolm Knowles, andragogy's most famous proponent, argued that adults were self-directed, problem-solving learners whose life experience constituted a significant learning resource" (Bartle, 2008, p. 1). In andragogy the role of the educator is more of a facilitator and the adult learner takes an active role in their education. Knowles developed the following set of assumptions that described the adult learner: they are self-directed; their life experiences become a learning resource; adults learn because they are motivated by what they need to know; they focus on problem-solving; and they have internal motivation to learn. Therefore, the relationship is one based on respect and collaboration and the teacher is more of a coach and embraces a learner-centered approach to teaching (Bartle, 2008). It is important to note that adult learners may be resistant to change and often have to balance their time between work, family, and school. One must also consider that each individual is unique and has different needs (Bastable, 2003).

> Knowles (1980) called upon educators to employ a seven step process in order to implement and capitalize upon the assumptions of andragogy. These steps included creating a cooperative learning climate; planning goals mutually; diagnosing learner needs and interests; helping learners to formulate learning objectives based on their needs and individual interests; designing sequential activities to achieve these objectives; carrying out the design to meet objectives with selected methods, materials, and resources; and evaluating the quality of the learning experience for the learner that included reassessing needs for continued learning. (Blondy, 2007, p. 117)

Educators can use these seven steps as a guide when developing educational offerings to the adult learner. It might not be possible to follow each of the seven steps but educators should think about how they can best meet the needs of the adult learner.

It is interesting to note that there has been some criticism of the use of andragogy because it was based mostly on observation and assumptions and not on empirical research. Thus research should be conducted on the use of andragogy and the principles of the adult learner. Therefore, educators must take many things into account when teaching adult students and find a balance between teaching and facilitating.

SUMMARY

In summary, philosophical beliefs and educational theory are utilized by educators to develop their own personal philosophy. Curricula frameworks are influenced by philosophical beliefs and vary among academic settings. Educational theories are selected based on their congruency with the philosophy and mission of the academic setting. Having knowledge of the various philosophical and theories will guide educators in the development of teaching and learning strategies for the adult learner.

DISCUSSION QUESTIONS

1. Compare and contrast the differences among idealism, essentialism, and realism
2. Describe the differences between the behaviorist and humanistic theories.
3. How are nurse educators influenced by moral and social theories?

4. Discuss critical social theory and education.
5. Describe the five main assumptions of Malcolm Knowles's theory of the adult learner.

SUGGESTED LEARNING ACTIVITIES

▪ Develop a lecture or presentation utilizing Knowles' principles of the adult learner.
▪ Conduct an in-depth review of the literature on one of the educational philosophies and one of the educational theories discussed in this chapter.

REFERENCES

Read more: http://www.experiment-resources.com/what-is-a-paradigm.html# ixzz1UHw42tNp.

Bartle, M. (2008). Andragogy. *Andragogy–Research Starters Education*, 1.

Bastable, S. (2003). Nurse as educator: Principles of teaching and learning for nursing practice. Sudbury, MA: Jones and Bartlett.

Billings, D. M., & Halstead, J. A. (2009). *Teaching in nursing: A guide for faculty* (3rd ed.). Philadelphia, PA: W.B. Saunders.

Blondy, L. (2007). Evaluation and application of andragogical assumptions to the adult online learning environment. *Journal of Interactive Online Learning, 6*(2), 116–130. Retrieved from Interactive Online Learning www.ncolr.org/jiol.

Brandon, A., & All, A. (2010). Constructivism theory analysis and application to curricula. *Nursing Education Perspectives, 31*(2), 89–92.

DeCarvalho, R. (1991). The humanistic paradigm in education. *The Humanistic Psychologist, 19*(1), 88–104.

Driscoll, M. P. (2000). *Psychology of learning for instruction* (2nd ed.). Boston, MA: Allyn and Bacon.

Eddy, J. (2002). Moving to a learner centered approach benefits students. *Teaching Matters* (6) 1, 7, Retrieved from www.cte.ku.edu/resources/ctePublications/ newsletters/.../index.shtml.

Eucken, R., & Phelps, M. (1880). Realism–Idealism. In R. Eucken, M. Phelps (Eds.), *The fundamental concepts of modern philosophic thought, critically and historically considered* (pp. 258–270). D Appleton & Company. doi:10.1037/12833-012.

Freire, P. (1972) Pedagogy of the Oppressed, Harmondsworth: Penguin.

Kretchmar, J. (2008). Social learning theory. Social learning theory–Research starters education, 1. Retrieved from EBSCOhost.

Li, Z. (2007). Supporting humanistic learning experiences through learning with technology. *International Journal of Learning, 13*(11), 131–136.

Meleis, A. (2007). Theoretical nursing development and progress (4th ed). Philadelphia: Lippincott, Williams, and Wilkins.

Milheim, K. L. (2011). The role of adult education philosophy in facilitating the online classroom. *Adult Learning, 22*(2), 24.

Mooney, M., & Nolan, L. (2006). A critique of Freire's perspective on critical social theory in nursing education. *Nurse Education Today, 26,* 240–244.

Shuttleworth, M. (2008). What is a paradigm?. Retrieved 20 Aug. 2012 from Experiment Resources: http://www.experiment-resources.com/what-is-a-paradigm.htmlRead more.

Smith, T. (2009). Aristotle & Realism. *Aristotle & Realism—Research Starters Education,* 1–6. Retrieved from EBSCOhost.

Stanley, M. C., & Dougherty, J. P. (2010). Nursing education model. A paradigm shift in nursing education: A new model. *Nursing Education Perspectives, 31*(6), 378–380. doi:10.1043/1536-5026-31.6.378.

Tabak, N., Adi, L., & Eherenfeld, M. (2003). A philosophy underlying excellence in teaching. *Nursing Philosophy, 4*(3), 249. Retrieved from EBSCOhost.

Uys, L. R., & Gwele, N. S. (2005). *Curriculum development in nursing: Process and innovations.* New York, NY: Routledge.

ADDITIONAL READINGS

Leonard, D. C. (2002). *Learning theories A to Z.* London: Greenwood.

Saulnier, B. M., Landry, J. P., Longenecker, J. E., & Wagner, T. A. (2008). From teaching to learning: Learner-centered teaching and assessment in information systems education. *Journal of Information Systems Education, 19*(2), 169–174. Retrieved from EBSCOhost.

CHAPTER 7

Learning Styles

"Never discourage anyone . . . who continually makes progress,
no matter how slow."

　　—PLATO

OBJECTIVES

After reading this chapter the reader will be able to:
- Identify auditory, visual, and kinetic teaching strategies
- Discuss cultural, generational, and gender issues
- Identify key components of David Kolb's model
- Discuss other learning style models
- Understand importance of utilizing a self-assessment of learning styles for self and students
- Identify online resources for examples of tools used to identify learning styles

INTRODUCTION

Learning is a unique experience for each person. Many factors contribute to how a person learns and although learning takes place in a multifaceted way most learners have a preferred learning style. In this chapter an overview of learning styles, cultural, gender, and generational issues and their significance in the teaching and learning experience will be discussed.

LEARNING STYLES

There are many different learning styles and a plethora of literature on learners and how they learn (Kolb, 1984, 1981; Minter, 2011). *"Learning style* refers to the ways individuals process information" (Guild & Garger, 1998, as cited in Bastable, 2003, p. 93). Learning styles are often classified as auditory, visual, and kinesthetic or tactile. An auditory learner will learn best when listening to a lecture, video, or recording. A visual learner will learn best when reading, taking notes, and looking at PowerPoints and videos. A kinesthetic or "hands on" learner will learn best when participating in a simulation or role play. Nurse educators need to be knowledgeable about learning styles and how they should be utilized when creating a positive educational environment (Kolb, 1984). As a new nurse educator you will also need to know your preferred style of learning, which will help you to better understand your students' specific educational needs (Bastable, 2003). Because typical classrooms are comprised of a diverse group of learners it is not possible to teach to just one style of learning. Therefore, educators should utilize a variety of teaching and learning strategies in the classroom to enhance the learning of all students. For example, for students who are visual learners the use of PowerPoints and visual aids should be utilized. Auditory learners will benefit from the use of lecture, DVDs, and podcasts. For tactile learners the use of simulation and hands-on experiences will enhance their learning. It is important to note that although there is often a predominant style of learning, students learn in a variety of ways. Students should be aware of their own learning styles because this will help them to be successful in their educational journey. There are a multitude of self-assessment tools on learning styles that can help to identify preferred learning style. Learners may then utilize this information to enhance their educational experience. Based on learning styles you can help students to set up specific plans to help them be successful. For example, some students find it very helpful to record lectures so that they can listen to them multiple times to reinforce information. As the teacher you must also decide if you are comfortable having a student tape your lecture. This is something you should discuss with your students so that there are no misunderstandings. There may be times, such as during test reviews, that tape recording is not allowed. You should also remind students that the recording is for their personal use and not to be posted on the internet or used for any other purposes (Learning Styles Online, 2011). There are many different ways to enhance learning and the use of technology in education will be discussed in Chapter 9.

Bastable (2003) discusses the six principles of learning style which include: identification of teaching and learning styles by teachers and students; teachers must try not to teach to only their preferred style; teachers should help students identify their own styles; teachers should utilize students' preferred styles; students should embrace other styles; and teachers should create and utilize each different style and modality.

KOLB's Learning Styles

There is a plethora of information that can be found in the literature on learning styles and David Kolb developed one of the most well known models. Kolb's model is based on experiential learning theory and includes four types of learning stages and four basic types of learning styles. The model is often depicted as a circle (see Figure 7.1), which identifies the learning cycle and includes concrete experience, reflective observation, abstract conceptualization, and active experimentation. It is the uniqueness of the learning experience to individual learners that results in a particular learning style.

According to Kolb, the learning process has two main dimensions. The first reaches from abstract conceptualization to concrete experience, and the second reaches from active experimentation to reflective observation. Kolb's learning style model says that the concrete experience and abstract conceptualization explains how the person perceives the knowledge, and the reflective observation and active experimentation explains how the person integrates the knowledge (Kaya, Özabacı, Tezel, 2009, p. 12).

The four learning styles identified by Kolb (1984) are diverger, assimilator, converger, and accommodator. The diverger is a concrete learner and likes to reflect upon situations and is usually very creative. The converger is an abstract thinker and prefers to analyze a situation and examine it from a logical perspective. Convergers are known as the "thinkers" and also are hands-on learners who prefer active experimentation. The assimilator is also an abstract thinker and, similar to the diverger, prefers reflective observation. Accommodators are concrete learners who also embrace active experimentation (Kaya et al., 2009; Kolb, 1984; Halsted, 2007). Being knowledgeable about these learning styles can help you to develop teaching and learning strategies that accommodate each one of these learning styles. Strategies that may be used with divergers include direct explanations and acting as a motivator. For convergers, allow them to problem solve and act more as a

FIGURE 7.1
LEARNING STYLES MODEL

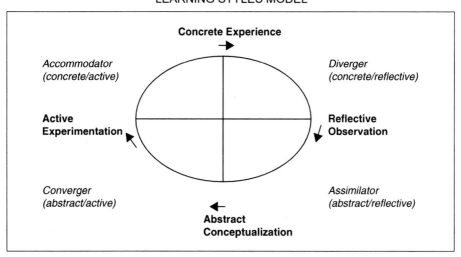

Adapted from Kolb's Learning Styles Model (1984). *Experiential learning: Experience as the source of learning and development* (1st ed.). Englewood Cliffs, NJ: Prentice Hall.

facilitator. For assimilators, teach in logical format and serve as an expert. For accommodators provide opportunities for hands-on learning activities that are well organized. Although not included in this book, there is a learning style inventory that was developed by Kolb (1984) that may be purchased and administered to students in order to identify preferred learning styles.

Models and Learning Styles

There is a vast array of literature on learning styles and learning style models. The following section will provide an overview of several well known models. The Myers-Briggs Type Indicator was developed from Carl Jung's theories on learning. Learners are classified as extraverts/introverts, sensors/intuitors, thinkers/feelers, judges/perceivers. (Felder, 1996; Personality-Power for everyday living.com, 2011).

The Herrmann Brain Dominance Instrument (HBDI) classifies learners according to brain dominance and includes four quadrants of the left and right brain. Learners classified as quadrant A are left-brain cerebral thinkers who are logical and analytical. Quadrant B thinkers are left-brain limbic thinkers who are sequential thinkers and detail oriented. Quadrant C thinkers are right-brain limbic thinkers who are emotional, sensory, and kinesthetic learners. Quadrant D thinkers are right-brain cerebral thinkers and are holistic and visual learners (Felder, 1996).

Another model was developed by Felder and Silverman (1988) for engineering students but can be applied to any learner. The Felder-Silverman learning style model classifies students as:

- *sensing learners* (concrete, practical, oriented toward facts and procedures) or *intuitive learners* (conceptual, innovative, oriented toward theories and meanings);
- *visual learners* (prefer visual representations of presented material—pictures, diagrams, flow charts) or *verbal learners* (prefer written and spoken explanations);
- *inductive learners* (prefer presentations that proceed from the specific to the general) or *deductive learners* (prefer presentations that go from the general to the specific);
- *active learners* (learn by trying things out, working with others) or *reflective learners* (learn by thinking things through, working alone);
- *sequential learners* (linear, orderly, learn in small incremental steps) or *global learners* (holistic, systems thinkers, learn in large leaps). (Felder, 1996, p. 220)

Models of learning and instruments that identify learning style preferences should be utilized by educators so that they can best meet the learning needs of their students. Utilizing a variety of teaching and learning strategies will create a learning environment that is conducive to all. Helping students to identify their learning style preference will enable them to be successful in their academic journey.

CULTURAL, GENERATIONAL, AND GENDER ISSUES

There are many factors that influence the way a student learns. Today most classrooms are diverse and comprised of students from a variety of backgrounds, which include ethnicity, culture, religion, gender, and age. These students often face greater challenges and may often feel isolated and misunderstood. As a nurse educator you will need to have a broad knowledge base of various cultures and address their learning needs on an individual basis.

Cultural issues greatly impact the learning environment and while it is impossible to know all cultures it is important to try to understand and facilitate learning of all the students in the class. Nursing programs are demanding for most students and an even greater challenge for students from different backgrounds. There are multiple areas that lend themselves to misinterpretation or difficult situations. One example is eye contact, which is revered in American and European cultures but may be considered disrespectful in Asian cultures and inappropriate between male and females in Muslim cultures. If faculty are not cognizant of this they may feel students are being disrespectful to them. Another issue is touching, which in many cultures and religions is taboo even in the form of a handshake. Students who have been taught in other countries will most likely have a different educational experience (Galanti, 2008; Jeffreys, 2010). For example, in some African countries, testing and evaluation of learning is done in the form of essays so when faced with a multiple choice test the students may not do well. Another issue is communication. This includes verbal and written communication (Andrews & Boyle, 2008; Giger & Davidhizer, 2008). Bednarz, Schim, and Doorenbos (2010) posit that one of the greatest cultural challenges in education is communication between students and faculty.

According to Bednarz et al. (2010):

> Language is the main mode of communication between nursing instructor and student; however, whether it is the spoken word or written work, language often can become a major stumbling block. Language issues become even more complex when faculty members and students have different backgrounds and speak different languages or dialects. (p. 257)

As an educator you will need to clearly articulate both written and verbal forms of communication. This is especially true in nursing because in addition to everything else students must learn all the new medical terms and jargon specific to the medical profession. Words and phrases may take on different meaning depending on one's frame of reference. You should serve as a role model for your students and help them to understand the terminology. Students need to understand your spoken voice, non-verbal communication, lectures, directions, instructions, syllabus, written work, and classroom etiquette. ESL (English as a second language) students may need accommodations so that they are not put at a disadvantage due to their language barrier.

Writing assignments are especially difficult and many students may write as they speak because they have not learned how to write an academic paper. Of course, you cannot possibly teach all of your students how to write but most educational settings have programs already in place to support students so you just need to be able to recognize and refer students who require these services.

"Instructors who were culturally aware and supportive were seen as primary and necessary resources for students in all studies" (Starr, 2009, p. 485). Instructor and student support measures include: mentoring, role modeling, tutoring, student clubs, peer support, and ethnic clubs (Starr, 2009).

Bednarz et al. (2010) found that:

> Cultural variations in approaches to academic work have been widely reported. Whereas the American higher education system places high value on independent thought and solo performance, students from many other cultures are taught to value work sharing and helping the whole group to achieve. (p. 258)

At times students may commit breaches of academic integrity because of cultural misunderstandings. It is important to be clear about expectations and issues of academic integrity because often students do not realize they are cheating when they are helping their fellow classmates because this was the norm back in their country.

Minority students are faced with many barriers to success in a nursing program. Some barriers relate to students' personal family situations where they must continue to provide financial support, or their families may lack understanding of the time and commitment required to be successful. In addition, there may be a feeling of academic inadequacy by the nursing students and struggles with language, racism, and isolation (Flynn, Brown, Johnson, & Rodger 2011). "According to Banks (1993), cultural conflicts occur in the classrooms because the personal/cultural knowledge that students of diverse cultures bring to the learning process is inconsistent with traditional school knowledge and with teachers' personal culture knowledge" (as cited in Leonard, 2006 p. 88). Adapting a caring curriculum may address some of these issues.

The caring curriculum has been described as follows:

> Bevis and Watson (1989) proposed that a caring curriculum is based on a position of human freedom, echoing nursing's traditional humanistic, existential philosophy. Educational principles of the caring curriculum (e.g., addressing wholeness, health, and healing; exhibiting self-respect and self-care; engaging with students in a moral, scientific manner) are well accepted. (as cited in Evans, 2004, p. 221)

The caring curriculum can foster positive relationships between faculty and students. "Through caring dialogue, faculty can role model supports for those different from themselves and integrate cultural concepts into daily classroom and testing activities" (Evans, 2004, p. 224). The application of this theory can be utilized in all educational settings, especially with minority nurses. It is challenging for all students to complete a nursing program and a caring curriculum can be beneficial to all students.

There are many ways faculty can develop in order to teach in a culturally congruent manner. Cultural competence is something that is continually developed as the educator becomes more knowledgeable about different cultures and practices. A good place to start is to reflect and analyze personal beliefs. Jeffreys (2010) recommends that nurse educators complete a self-assessment of their cultural values and beliefs (CVB). They can then use the results of this assessment to identify areas that need to be improved. "After self-assessment, nurse educators who have not had optimal shares positive views, values, beliefs, and experiences with students should make a concerted effort to do so" (Jeffreys, 2010, p. 124). As a nurse educator you have a dual role in regards to cultural competence; one is to self-develop and become culturally competent and the other is to help students to become culturally competent. You also need to be a role model for providing culturally congruent care to all patients.

GENDER ISSUES

Gender issues include both the female and male populations. Nursing is a predominately female profession and for many years has been viewed as an oppressed group. However, in recent years there has been a shift and nurses have become more empowered. Another issue in nursing is male students who comprise about 5.8% of the total nursing population. Male nursing students may feel unwelcome or out of place. They have also been subject to stereotyping and many people assume males are not as caring or nurturing as females.

Oppressed Groups

As previous discussed in chapter 6 Freire has written extensively critical social theory and oppressed groups. Mooney and Nolan (2006) wrote a critique of Freire's work on critical social theory in nursing education and the following is a synopsis of their critique. Freire's goal was to empower students and help students to be autonomous. According to Freire, praxis was the key to liberation. Critical praxis involves synchronized reflection and action. This provides a basis for how one comes to know and guides one toward liberation. Oppression in nursing has been fostered by the use of the biomedical model and educators who continued to use traditional approaches to education. Oppression can lead to aggression and complaint that is directed within the group instead of at the oppressors. "Freire (1972) noted that the education process could act as a tool for conformity or an instrument for liberation and promoted an education based on liberation, whereby individuals are empowered through critical examination of their reality" (as cited in Mooney & Nolan,

2006, p. 241). The role of the educator is key to this process. The educator must be reflective and communicative to foster students' growth and enable students to critically think and become independent in their thoughts. The educators must also become empowered so that they can enable their students to become empowered. Developing educational programs that have been influenced by Freire can help nursing achieve this goal. Professional growth and development can be realized through the use of critical social theory. Nursing must continue to grow and further define its body of knowledge in order to overcome prejudices that have existed in the past. Emancipation and knowledge development can be achieved with critical engagement. Nurse educators can help to empower nurses through their mentoring, guidance, leadership, and support in the educational setting.

Traditionally males in nursing have been stereotyped as being effeminate or less caring. This has resulted in a disproportionately low number of male nurses. "According to traditional societal stereotypes, men have been viewed as less caring individuals. Characteristics traditionally attributed to women include caring, compassion, and nurturing" (Ierardi, Fitzgerald, & Holland, 2010, p. 215). The results of a recent qualitative study by Ierardi et al. (2010) identified four major themes in regards to males in nursing. The four themes were: "wanting to care for others, leaving another career or vocation to pursue nursing, having a positive experience in the nursing program, and being mistaken for physicians" (p. 216). The researchers were surprised that this sample of male nurses, contrary to what has been stated in the literature, had found their program and instructors positive and supportive. In an earlier study Smith (2006) concluded that: male nurses would benefit from a support group; issues regarding female patients' refusal to be treated by a male nurse should be explored; language in textbooks and classrooms should represent male and female students; and male mentoring programs should be developed. Faculty need to take a proactive approach in facilitating learning in diverse student populations.

GENERATIONAL ISSUES

Many higher education settings have students from a variety of ages and generations. This is also a factor that faculty must consider when planning courses, learning activities, lectures, and evaluations. Throughout the years education has changed dramatically especially in the area of technology. Most higher education classrooms today will be comprised of the several generations which include Millennials who were born between 1979–2000, the Generation Xers born between 1965–1978, and the Baby Boomers from 1947–1964 (Takase, Maude, & Manias, 2006). These groups come with very different foundational learning and life experiences. The traditional nursing student who attends directly from high school comprises less than half of your class. The other half may come from any one of the generations and this may be a first or second career. Technology can be a major obstacle for the Baby Boomers and some Generation Xers but you can never assume that Millenials are computer literate. Baby Boomers have been described as learners who are serious, determined, value respect, and value the role of the teacher. They do not like group work and prefer to work independently. They are often concrete learners and do best when expectations are clearly defined. Generation Xers have been describes as learners who prefer to learn in innovative and creative ways. They also value their free time and strive to seek a balance between school, work, and leisure. The Millenials expect technology and creativity in the classroom. They are used to learning at a fast pace with innovative strategies and will make their needs known. They also enjoy group work.

SUMMARY

There are seven common learning style preferences that have been identified. They include: visual, aural, verbal, physical, logical, social, and solitary. A visual learner prefers to learn by sight. Activities such as reading, looking at pictures, viewing PowerPoints and images will help this type of student to learn. An aural learner learns best through hearing. Activities such as listening to lectures, recording lectures, audio books, and music will facilitate learning.

A verbal learner learns through reading words and listening to speakers. A physical learner requires hands-on or kinesthetic activities. Participating in experiments, role-playing, and simulation are recommended. A logical learner needs concrete information and will do well in mathematics. A social learner enjoys group work such as case studies, group projects, and study groups. A solitary learner enjoys working alone and feels more comfortable in quiet situations. Completing individual assignments will work best for this type of learner.

This chapter focused on learning styles and types of learners. An overview of four models was presented. Challenges related to culture, gender, and generation were discussed.

Specific learning styles and related teaching strategies were also addressed.

DISCUSSION QUESTIONS

1. Discuss the seven types of learning styles and a teaching strategy for each one.
2. Compare and contrast the four learning style models that were presented in this chapter.
3. Describe how learning styles influence your teaching style.
4. Identify barriers to learning related to cultural, gender, and generational issues.
5. Discuss the four main types of learner style preferences in Kolb's model.

SUGGESTED LEARNING ACTIVITIES

- Complete a learning style assessment online at: people.usd.edu/~bwjames/ tut/learning-style/ or www.learning-styles-online.com/overview/.
- Prepare a ten-minute presentation on a topic of your choice and develop teaching and learning strategies based on two different styles of learning models that you read about in this chapter.
- Conduct a review of the literature on learning style models and learning styles and write a ten-page essay.

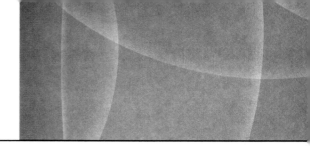

Reflection

RHONDA BROGDON, DNP, MSN, MBA, RN

I HAVE WORKED IN ACADEME FOR six years as a nurse educator. During this time, I have faced challenges that have fostered my professional growth, my commitment to my university's expectations of me as faculty member, and my accountability in maintaining high standards in academia. I have learned that when I teach my students about time management and prioritization, utilizing this skill is just as crucial for me. Transitioning from bedside nursing into academia included some "different" yet "similar" attributes: Just like the patients were my responsibility in bedside nursing, the students are my responsibility in academe. I needed to be aware of their learning styles, in order to facilitate their understanding. I needed to learn about different teaching techniques and learning styles of students to manage a range of learning styles to foster students' understanding of the content I was presenting.

I have learned as an educator that it is very important to network within and outside your institution. For example, students today are met with test-taking problems and anxiety. Knowing what resources are available on your campus and community helps you to direct these anxious students to the appropriate person or organization.

I have also learned that the university's faculty handbook is a vital component to knowing your role as a faculty member. This is definitely one book you should not lay aside. It has helped me tremendously in understanding the expectations the university has of me. The university handbook articulates exactly what is expected of me with regard to teaching, scholarship, and service. While the handbook is an indispensible guide for new faculty, being assigned a faculty mentor is even more valuable in guiding you in the process of what is important in these areas, especially when it comes to tenure and promotion.

With regards to service, participation in university activities such as open houses, health fairs, and scholarship interviews is very helpful. Also, it is important to participate in activities that support the community, such as flu shot administrations, heart walks, screenings (blood pressure); moreover, your professional service to your department is also significant such as serving departmental committees and what you do for your professional advancement such as attending publication workshops and tenure/ promotion workshops. Scholarship activities could include being an abstract reviewer or submitting a research or capstone project, professional honor societies, grant writing, in addition to presenting at educational conferences. In teaching, make sure you keep track of what courses you teach each semester, the student number in each class, along with the semester and year. In addition, make sure that you keep all of your student evaluations for each semester. This is an important section when you begin to develop and compile your information for tenure and promotion.

I am not only a nurse educator. I am an advisor, designer and developer of curricula, and sometimes, a mother. I had no idea that my role in education would require so much and that I would take so much work home. You just don't teach and go home . . . you are constantly learning, growing, and modifying ways to facilitate learning to students. As a nurse educator, you are doing your best to keep your students on the right path to be successful in their professional and personal growth.

As a moderately experienced nurse educator, my advice to new nurse educators would be:

- First, take one day at a time. Try not to do everything at once . . . know your limits; time is priceless and lifelong treasure.
- Second, explore your internal and external motivators that will facilitate your nurse educator role.
- Third, maintain your clinical competence to facilitate learning for your students and importantly yourself.
- Fourth, remember, one teaching style does not work for everyone.
- Fifth, utilize your university and department handbooks.
- Sixth, don't be afraid to network and ask questions; it is how we learn, and lastly, "empower" yourself, you determine your success.

REFERENCES

Andrews, M., & Boyle, J. (2008). *Transcultural concepts in nursing care* (5th ed.). Philadelphia, PA: Wolters Kluwer & Lippincott.

Banks, James A., and Cherry Banks. 1993. Multicultural education: Issues and perspectives. 2nd edition. Boston: Allyn and Bacon

Banks, J. (1993). Approaches to multicultural curriculum reform. In J. Banks and C. Banks (Eds.), Multicultural education: Issues and perspectives. Boston: Allyn & Bacon.

Bastable, S. (2003). *Nurse as educator principles of teaching and learning for nurse practice* (2nd ed.). Sudbury, MA: Jones & Bartlett.

Bednarz, H., Schim, S., & Doorenbos, A. (2010). Cultural diversity in nursing education: Perils, pitfalls, and pearls. *Journal of Nursing Education, 49*(5), 253–260.

Bevis, E., & Watson, J. (1989). Towards a Caring Curriculum: A New Pedagogy for Nursing. New York: National League for Nursing.

Evans, B. C. (2004). Application of the caring curriculum to education of Hispanic/Latino and American Indian nursing students. *Journal of Nursing Education, 43*(5), 219–228.

Freire, P. (1972) Pedagogy of the Oppressed, Harmondsworth: Penguin.

Felder, R. (1996). Matters of style. *ASEE Prism, 6*(4), 18–23. Retrieved from www.ncsu.edu/felder-public/Papers/LS-Prism.htm.

Felder, R. M., & Silverman, L. K. (1988). Learning and Teaching Styles in Engineering Education, Engr. Education, *78*(7), 674–681.

Flynn, S., Brown, J., Johnson, A., & Rodger, S. (2011). Barriers to education for the marginalized adult learner. *Alberta Journal of Educational Research, 57*(1), 43–58.

Galanti, G. A. (2008). *Caring for patients from different cultures* (4th ed.). Philadelphia, PA: University of Pennsylvania Press.

Giger, J., & Davidhizar, R. (2008). *Transcultural nursing: Assessment & intervention* (5th ed.). St. Louis, MO: Mosby/Elsevier.

Guild, P., & Garger, S. (1998). Marching to Different Drummers. 2nd edition. Published by the Association for Supervision and Curriculum Development (Alexandria, VA).

Ierardi, J. A., Fitzgerald, D. A., & Holland, D. T. (2010). Exploring male students' educational experiences in an associate degree nursing program. *Journal of Nursing Education, 49*(4), 215–218.

Jeffreys, M. (2010). *Teaching cultural competence in nursing and in health care* (2nd ed.). New York, NY: Springer.

Kaya, F., Özabacı, N., & Tezel, Ö. (2009). Investigating primary school second grade students' learning styles according to the Kolb learning style model in terms of demographic variables. *Journal of Turkish Science Education (TUSED), 6*(1), 11–25.

Kolb, D. A. (1984). *Experiential learning: Experience as the source of learning and development.* Englewood Cliffs, NJ: Prentice Hall.

Kolb, D. A. (1981). Learning styles and disciplinary differences. In A. W. Chickering & Associates (Eds.), *The modern American college: Responding to the new realities of diverse students and a changing society* (pp. 232–255). San Francisco: Jossey-Bass.

Learning Styles Online.com. (2011). Overview of learning styles. Retrieved from www.learning-styles-online.com/overview.

Leonard, T. (2006). Exploring diversity in nursing education: Research findings. *Journal of Cultural Diversity, 13*(2), 87–96.

Minter, R. L. (2011). The learning theory jungle. *Journal of College Teaching & Learning, 8*(6), 7–15.

Mooney, M., & Nolan, L. (2006). A critique of Freire's perspective on critical social theory in nursing education. Nurse Education Today, 26, 240–244.

Personality-Power for everyday living.com. (2011). Retrieved from www.personality-power-for-everyday-living.com/learning-style-inveChicago/Turabian:Author-Date.

Smith, J. (2006). Exploring the challenges for nontraditional male students transitioning into a nursing program. *Journal of Nursing Education, 45*(7), 263–269.

Starr, K. (2009). Nursing education challenges: Students with English as an additional language. *Journal of Nursing Education, 48*(9), 478–487.

Takase, M., Maude, P., & Manias, E. (2006). Role discrepancy: Is it a common problem among nurses? Journal of Advanced Nursing, *54*(6), 751–759.

ADDITIONAL READINGS

Hermann, J. (2008). *Creative teaching strategies for the nurse educator.* Philadelphia, PA: Davis Company.

Jeffreys, M. R. (2004). *Nursing student retention: Understanding the process and making a difference.* New York, NY: Springer.

CHAPTER 8

Course Development

"The essence of teaching is to make learning contagious, to have one idea spark another."

—MARY COLLINS

OBJECTIVES

After reading this chapter, the reader will be able to
- Develop a course syllabus
- Understand the difference between goals, objectives, and learning outcomes
- Identify key areas of course planning
- Discuss teaching and learning strategies
- Select required and supplemental material
- Grade assignments
- Compare theory and clinical teaching

INTRODUCTION

This chapter will focus on the components of developing and teaching both theory and clinical courses. Planning and developing a course is time consuming and requires much thought and preparation. One of the most important components is the course syllabus, which is considered a contract between you and your students. Many academic settings have templates for their faculty to follow. These may include standardized course descriptions and learning objectives. Another big challenge is the organization and timing of lectures within the course.

Designing and planning your course from the big picture to the smallest detail will help you to run your course in a logical and timely fashion.

DEVELOPING A COURSE SYLLABUS

The course syllabus is a document that is created either individually or collaboratively and is required for every course taught in an academic setting. Course syllabi come in different formats but most of them have similar components. When developing a course syllabus it is important to follow the guidelines of the particular academic setting. For example, if templates are mandatory, they must be utilized. Even when a specific template is not required, often there is an accepted format to use when constructing a syllabus. These may vary among settings (see Exhibit 8.1). It is important to note that the syllabus is a legal contract between the faculty and the students and must be adhered to by both parties (Thompson, 2007).

The major components of the course syllabus include:

- Course information
- Course description
- Instructor information
- Course objectives/learning outcomes
- Textbooks
- Required and supplemental readings
- Materials
- Assignments and guidelines and rubrics
- Policies for attendance and participation
- Clinical policies for a clinical course
- Evaluation methods and grading policies
- Academic integrity
- Support services
- Course schedule/weekly outline/assignments

Creating a course syllabus for the first time can be a daunting task so be sure to seek guidance from your faculty colleagues and mentor. If the course was taught previously, you may use a copy of the old syllabus as a guide when creating your own. If several sections of the same course are being taught by different faculty, it is a good idea to collaborate with them and create a standard course syllabus. Adhering to this practice reduces the tendency for students to feel that one section is better than another section or one group is required to do more work than another group taking a different section of the same course. In some settings, course syllabi are approved by the curriculum committee.

While it is important to follow the guidelines in your setting, the following are some standard guidelines:

1. Give each student a printed or electronic copy of the syllabus on the first day of the course.
2. Encourage students to use the syllabus as a roadmap for the course and to refer to it frequently throughout the semester.

EXHIBIT 8.1

Sample Course Syllabus Template

University x
COURSE OVERVIEW/CLINICAL

COURSE NUMBER:	NUR _____
COURSE TITLE:	
CREDITS/HOURS:	2 credits/90 hours
PLACEMENT IN CURRICULUM:	Fall, Spring, Summer
PREREQUISITES:	NUR _____, NUR _____, NUR _____
COREQUISITES:	NUR 4XX, NUR 4XX, NUR 4XX, NUR 4XX
FACULTY:	Mary Smith, PhD, RN
	Assistant Professor of Nursing
	Office Location:
	Phone: 900-333-22XX
	Email: msmith@universityx.com
	Office Hours
TERM:	Fall _____
CATALOG DESCRIPTION:	_____

STUDENT LEARNING OUTCOMES/COURSE OUTCOMES:

At the completion of this course, the student will achieve the following identified course objectives: (list learning objectives and expected outcomes)

1. Synthesize concepts and theories as evidenced by:

    a. _____

    b. _____

    c. _____

TEACHING STRATEGIES:

Pre/post conferences
Formal Papers

(continued)

EXHIBIT 8.1

Sample Course Syllabus Template **(continued)**

EVALUATION METHODS/LEARNING OUTCOMES

- Formative Evaluation   Objectives 1–5
- Summative Evaluation   Objectives 1–5
- Weekly assessments, journals, and
  care plans   Objectives 1–5

REQUIRED REFERENCES:

Author (year)
Author (year)

CLINICAL EVALUATIONS

There will be a formative (mid-term) and summative (final) clinical evaluation. When meeting the clinical instructor for formative and summative evaluations, the student may bring a copy of the clinical evaluation tool as a self-assessment work sheet. The student must document where the clinical instructor can find evidence that he/she have met, or is working toward each clinical objective.

PRE CONFERENCE

POST-CONFERENCE

Written Assignments

All written papers must follow APA format.

3. Verbally review the course syllabus and expectations on the first day of class.
4. Be certain there are no errors in the syllabus because once you post and review the syllabus it is considered the binding copy. So it is highly recommended to have someone review it before you post it. If you do notice an error after it has been posted, you should consult with the administration at your academic setting for guidance on how to proceed.
5. Adhere to your syllabus. For example, if you say that students will lose points for being late or absent or not participating you need to be consistent with every student.
6. Do not change assignments or grading policies once the syllabus has been posted and reviewed with students; you must follow your syllabus exactly as it is stated.

A well developed syllabus provides many advantages for both faculty and students:

1. It can make your job as faculty easier because a well developed syllabus outlines the course expectations and both student and faculty responsibilities. There is less chance for misunderstandings.
2. It provides students with a clear set of expectations and faculty with a plan that is consistent throughout the semester.
3. It helps to avoid both legal and academic problems.

GOALS, OBJECTIVES, AND LEARNING OUTCOMES

When developing a course, faculty must consider the purpose of the course and the expected goals, objectives, and outcomes. *Goals* are broad statements about the course and overall learning outcomes. "A *goal* is the final outcome of what is achieved at the end of the teaching-learning process. Goals are global and broad in nature; they serve as long-term targets for both the learner and the teacher" (Bastable, 2003, p. 312). An example of a goal is *the learner will apply concepts in nursing theory and practice*. *Objectives* are more specific and concise statements that relate to the goals and the learning outcomes. "Objectives must be achieved before the goal can be reached. They must be observable and measureable to be able to determine whether they have been met by the learner" (Bastable, 2003, p. 321). An example of a well written objective is: At the end of this class *the learner will be able to identify the difference between embolic and hemorrhagic strokes*. "Together, objectives and goals form a map that provides directions (objectives) as to how to arrive at a particular destination (goal)" (Bastable, 2003, p. 321).

The three major categories of behavioral objectives are the domains of cognitive, affective, and psychomotor. They identify the students' expected achievement of knowledge, skills, and attitudes upon completing the course work.

■ Cognitive objectives relate to thinking and acquisition of empirical knowledge. They reflect the student's values or beliefs that have changed because of learning that took place.
■ Affective objectives relate to caring beliefs and thoughts and feelings about a topic.
■ Psychomotor objectives relate to tasks and behavior related to skills acquisition.

Objectives should be measurable and attainable and often include all three domains. They relate more specifically to student performance and may reflect specific content. The statements should be brief and to the point. *Learning outcomes* are the specific achievement expected of the student at the end of the course. They reflect what the learner will achieve or know at the end of the course and are more student centered. Outcomes should contain action words and reflect the mission and philosophy of the program and the college or university. Issues related to poorly written objectives include; setting unrealistic goals, writing goals that are not measurable; and focusing on the instructor's role instead of the learner's expected outcomes (Bastable, 2003; University of Connecticut, 2011).

The following are some other factors to consider when developing goals and objectives:

- Target audience
- Purpose of course
- Content
- Expected student outcomes
- Expected skills to be achieved

There are many resources available on how to develop goals and objectives and the old adage "practice makes perfect" can guide your foray into this unchartered territory. It is helpful to have an experienced faculty member review your course objectives after you write your first draft. Eventually you will become proficient in developing your own course offerings.

Bloom's taxonomy (Bloom, 1956) often is used in developing learning objectives because it addresses the domains of learning and also increases in complexity. The six domains developed by Bloom are knowledge, comprehension, application, analysis, synthesis, and evaluation. Knowledge, the first level, relates to recall of basic facts. Knowledge-based objectives would include statements such as list, define, and select. The next level is comprehension and relates to understanding, comparing, and interpreting information acquired. Comprehension-level objectives would include statements such as explain, outline, compare, and contrast. Bloom's third level is application and relates to problem solving and utilizing new concepts. Application-level objective statements would include the words apply, construct, utilize, and identify. The fourth level is analysis and relates to making inferences and finding evidence. Analysis-level objectives statements would include the words analyze, evaluate, and examine. The fifth level is synthesis and relates to combining information or creating solutions. Synthesis-level objective statements would include the words formulate, predict, and theorize. The highest level is evaluation, which relates to judgments and validity of ideas. Evaluation-level objective statements would include words such as conclude, defend, and interpret (Bastable, 2003; Eber & Parker, 2007; UNNC, 2011).

These same principles utilized in objective creation for a course syllabus are applicable when developing presentations or continuing education courses. It is important to know your audience and their backgrounds so you can utilize the appropriate course objectives for your target audience. In 1999,

Dr. Lorin Anderson, a former student of Bloom's, revised the taxonomy to reflect teaching and learning more broadly and in response to advances in education that have taken place since Bloom developed the original taxonomy. The new terms are defined as:

▦ *Remembering*: Retrieving, recognizing, and recalling relevant knowledge from long-term memory.
▦ *Understanding*: Constructing meaning from oral, written, and graphic messages through interpreting, exemplifying, classifying, summarizing, inferring, comparing, and explaining.
▦ *Applying*: Carrying out or using a procedure through executing, or implementing.
▦ *Analyzing*: Breaking material into constituent parts, determining how the parts relate to one another and to an overall structure or purpose through differentiating, organizing, and attributing.
▦ *Evaluating*: Making judgments based on criteria and standards through checking and critiquing.
▦ *Creating*: Putting elements together to form a coherent or functional whole; reorganizing elements into a new pattern or structure through generating, planning, or producing (Anderson & Krathwohl, 2001, pp. 67–68).

Utilizing the domains in either the original or newer version of this taxonomy will help to guide you in the development of well developed, higher-order learning objectives that can be utilized with increasing complexity as students advance in their programs. Bloom's taxonomy is also utilized in developing assessment and evaluation tools and will be further discussed in Chapter 10.

COURSE PLANNING

One of the biggest challenges to new and even experienced faculty is planning courses and lectures. You have only a certain amount of time to meet goals and objectives, to present all the required content, and to evaluate learning outcomes. Organization and time management skills are extremely important and whether you are presenting a single course offering or a semester-long course you will need to plan accordingly so that your students can meet the goals, and achieve the course objectives and learning outcomes. It is helpful to use a daily, weekly, monthly, and even yearly planner to keep organized. Creating a course offering form (see Exhibit 8.2) is strongly recommended. This is an excellent way to ensure that topics are presented in timely fashion. Although it may be time consuming, it is well worth the effort. Eventually, you will have a wonderful resource of well developed course offerings. These can be used again and edited to reflect updated content or research.

There are several factors that will guide your course planning. The first is the type of course to be taught. If you are giving a presentation or continuing education course, you will be preparing one discrete course offering.

EXHIBIT 8.2

Course Offering—Sample

Topic: *Topic of presentation or course offering*
Goals: *List one or two goals*

Learning Objectives	Topical Outline	Time Allocation	Instructor	Teaching Methods
Include cognitive, affective, and psychomotor objectives	List the specific topics related to each objective. This should be done in the order of how you present your course	List amount of time to be spent on each topic	List the names of all instructors	List all teaching methods (e.g., lecture, video, role plays)

However, if you are teaching a course in an academic setting, you will be planning for the entire semester. Another is to allow for holidays when mapping out the semester. A third is to consider the extent of content to be covered in the course. Whether you are teaching one topic or an entire course, it is a good idea to list all the content that you want to include. A concept map or lesson plan can be helpful in determining specific content and time allocation for each topic. Time allocation can be especially tricky. Calculating time needed to teach desired content can be elusive, but there are several strategies that can help:

1. Practice or tape your presentation to determine how long the presentation will take. You never really know how long a presentation will take until you actually teach it. Every minute counts and each class must be carefully planned with specific time allocated for presenting all the content.
2. Build in extra time for each presentation to accommodate the teaching of content that might be more difficult to convey and to account for a variety of student learning styles. It is best not to rush students through a presentation,

so the more you practice the better you will be able to judge how much time you should spend on each topic.

3. Allow time for questions and answers. Some faculty allow time at the end of a lesson and others take questions during the entire lesson. You need to find a balance between pacing your presentation and allowing for questions and breaks. It is important to pace your presentation so that you do not talk too fast or too slow.

4. Plan for breaks if necessary: the average adult attention span is about 20 minutes. You can usually pick up cues from your students as to when they need a break. When students begin to fidget, yawn, or stop participating it is usually a good time to take a break. Planned breaks work well and should be allocated based on the length of the presentation. Some faculty ask the students about their preferences in regards to scheduling time for breaks. A good rule of thumb is 10 minutes for every hour.

5. Utilize a two-minute stretch, especially when teaching complex topics.

6. Pace your lecture/presentation. Place a watch or clock within easy view so you can keep track of the time. You have to find a balance between presenting too fast and presenting too slow.

All of these strategies are helpful to ensure the delivery of an effective class lecture. Becoming an expert presenter takes time and the more you practice the better you will become at delivering and teaching content in a specified amount of time. Having someone videotape you during a practice session can be extremely helpful as you can critique yourself before you actually teach the course. Although it may seem like a lot of work to become prepared, you most likely will be teaching the same or similar topics multiple times so the prep for teaching this first course will reap rewards in the long term.

COURSE CONTENT

Knowing something and teaching something are very different. As a nurse educator you will be teaching topics you know but this is not enough to ensure that you are an effective educator. Your goal is to become an expert in your topics. To achieve this goal will require spending time reading and researching all the topics you will be teaching to ensure that you have a broad knowledge base. In academic settings most faculty teach both theory and clinical courses in their area of expertise; to become "expert" you just need to continue expanding your knowledge base and keep up to date on current research, technology, and trends. There is a wealth of information in your textbooks, libraries, and the internet so you should have no trouble finding good resources. Furthermore, many textbooks come with excellent faculty resources and tools that can be adapted to your specific needs. Of course, you also need to adhere to the curriculum of your academic setting and be sure to include all content required of the curriculum and by licensing and accrediting agencies. Consulting with faculty who have taught the course previously is also helpful. Remember that the first time you teach a course will be the most difficult, but being prepared will help to ensure that all goes smoothly.

There are times when you will have to teach a totally new course about a topic with which you are not familiar. Tackling this challenge will take more preparation and planning but can be done. Ideally, you will have ample time to prepare for a new course. You will need to prepare in all the same ways as for other courses, but teaching a new topic requires more time learning about the content you will be teaching. Again, consulting with a faculty member who has previously taught the class or has team-taught the course can be helpful. Another strategy is to arrange for guest speakers who are expert on the topic to help shoulder some of the burden when dealing with highly complex material.

Preparing for a Clinical Course

Preparing for a clinical course is somewhat different than teaching a theory course. Preparing course material for this type of course is similar to the theory course but has different components. In this type of course the instruction is often more informal and done in small groups and on an individual basis. If you are an adjunct, the course syllabus and material may have been completed by the course coordinator. You will need to work closely with the theory instructor and the course coordinator as the students will be expected to apply theoretical concepts while caring for a variety of different patients during the course of the semester. Many theory and clinical courses are integrated and the students have to pass both components in order to pass both theory and clinical. A failure in either one will result in students retaking both courses. Depending on the level and type of course there will be specific learning objectives and clinical experiences that need to be accomplished by the end of the semester. This requires careful planning on the part of the clinical faculty so that all students have a similar experience.

Sometimes there is only one syllabus that includes both the theory and clinical components and other times the two components are developed as two separate syllabi. The main goal is to have course syllabi that clearly reflect what the students are expected to learn and achieve by the end of the semester.

COURSE COMPONENTS

Textbooks

Selecting a textbook is another important task of faculty and can be done in several ways. You may be expected to select your own textbook or this selection may be made by a faculty group. When you have a choice in textbook selection, you should preview several different textbooks to see which one best meets the needs of your course objectives. Book publishers send out complimentary desk copies of textbooks for faculty to review before adoption decisions for their course are made. Recommended textbooks and supplemental material should also be reviewed before adding them to your syllabus. Because no book can meet all of your course objectives, you will want to consider including supplemental material such as journal articles, library course reserves, DVDs, and other resources. As part of your weekly course outline you will need to assign specific chapters and supplemental material that students must complete before each class. Be sure to review all materials before assigning them to students. You should also be realistic when assigning weekly readings (Wolfe, 2004).

Evaluation and Grading Methods

Evaluation of student learning through the completion of homework, quizzes, tests, papers, case studies, care plans, and observation is another very important responsibility of the nurse educator. Evaluation methods are aimed at measuring the goals, objectives, and learning outcomes of the course. Because students possess different learning styles, it is best to use a variety of evaluation methods. The weekly course outline should list the evaluation methods and the list the date when each is due so that students may plan their time accordingly. Each evaluation method must be weighted in points or percentages that equal 100%. This information should be included in the course syllabus and cannot be changed once the syllabus is posted. However, if there is something that you feel must be changed, you should consult with the dean/chair on the policy for revising a course syllabus.

The following is an example of a weighted evaluation plan:

Quiz #1 = 20 points/percent   Scholarly paper = 20 points/percent
Quiz #2 = 20 points/percent   Final Exam = 25 points/percent
Case Study = 5 points/percent   Homework = 10 points/percent

There may be specific requirements for grading and evaluation that must be followed. For example, some schools require a certain percent of the evaluation to come from exams and a certain percent from written work. It is important to give students an opportunity to demonstrate their learning, and assignments and grading should be fair and balanced. When creating an assignment always consider how it relates to the course objectives and what outcomes you are hoping to measure. For writing assignments give specific guidelines including the use of APA and a grading rubric so that students know exactly what is expected. Many schools have writing centers where students can go to receive guidance on scholarly writing. Creating exams is challenging and you will need guidance from an experienced faculty mentor in this area. There are many wonderful resources that may be utilized when developing exams and writing test items that are valid and reliable. Some schools create exams as a committee or have a committee review your exam before it is administered to students. Exams may be graded by hand or on an electronic grading system. These systems grade exams and prepare an analysis of your exam with an item analysis for each question. This helps to identify problem areas and establish reliability and validity of test items. You can also do this by hand but it is very time consuming. Some faculty send students a test blueprint or study guide to help them prepare for their exams.

This is optional and there are proponents both for and against this practice. You will need to follow the specific policies of the school and do what you feel is best for you and your students.

Clinical courses are usually pass/fail and require a formative and summative evaluation to be completed that demonstrates that the student has met the course objectives. These forms may also be standardized and approved by the faculty to be used in all courses. Students must be made aware of their progress and early notification and formal meetings should take place with any student who is in danger of failing the course. It is important to keep detailed records and consult with administration regarding any concerns with student progress. Remember to always be fair and objective when evaluating student outcomes. Currently there is an emphasis on utilizing evidence-based practice when developing evaluation methods to evaluate student learning. It is important to utilize valid and reliable tools and complete them in a timely manner.

TEACHING AND LEARNING STRATEGIES

Another component of course planning is deciding which teaching and learning strategies to use to deliver your content. It is best to use a variety of methods in an effort to address the individual learning needs of a diverse group of students. Some of the most common teaching strategies include lectures, case studies, role playing, simulation, videos, PowerPoint presentations, use of anecdotes and stories, student presentations, guest speakers, discussion, and critical thinking exercises. Again the caveat is that specific objectives and outcomes must be related to all learning activities.

Beginning a new course with an ice breaker is a good idea to ease tension. There are many things you can do such as puzzles, games, and riddles. Another way to handle student introductions is to pair students together and have them ask each other questions such as their name, why they want to be a nurse, and to state a goal they have for the course. Then after you introduce yourself have each student introduce their partner to the class. This is a great way to welcome students and get to know you and their fellow classmates (Hermann, 2008).

The lecture method is still widely used and lends itself well to teaching complex topics. Lectures must be well planned and paced so that students remain interested. Combining the use of PowerPoints or some other type of visual aid will enhance the lecture. Encouraging student participation and interaction during the lecture will also keep it interesting. It is important to prepare lecture notes based on your course offering. You should never just sit in front of the room and read from the textbook or read word for word from a busy PowerPoint slide. You should be standing and moving around the room and engaging the students. It is helpful to intersperse some humor and real-life stories. Whenever possible your room should be arranged in an orderly and appealing fashion. PowerPoint presentations are commonly used by nurse educators and are a great tool. However, one major criticism is that the slides are too busy and contain too much information. PowerPoint presentations should enhance your lecture and discussions so remember "less is more"; including information as bullets with a few key words and graphics is best. Many textbooks have prepared PowerPoint presentations that can be edited for individual needs.

Group discussions and Socratic questioning (probing questions) are another great way to teach but only work if class size is not too large. Preparing a list of questions based on the assigned readings is good way to have a group discussion. You may want to assign specific questions or go around the room so that each student must participate in the discussion. In this method your role is more of a facilitator and while a rich and varied discussion is a wonderful way to learn you must also strive to maintain order and stay on the subject. If having a group discussion, a circle is best so if possible, request a room well in advance that will allow you to place desks or chairs in one big circle (Billings & Halstead, 2009).

Case studies in the form of group participation or small groups of student presentations are a great way to teach about disease processes and clinical applications. You will need to develop clear guidelines and expectations for student presentations. Humor is a great teaching tool but must be done in such a way as not to offend anyone and should also be used intermittently. Stories and anecdotes are also a good way to teach a lesson while keeping students very involved. Asking students to share their clinical experiences is a great way to relate clinical and theoretical components.

Audiovisual material can be used to teach part of a course or enhance a lecture or presentation. You may consider videos, CD ROMs, DVDs, posters, and online resources. There are also many interactive DVDs that promote critical thinking and students can work individually or in a group. Presentations may be video streamed or podcasts can be used. Technology and learning will be discussed in greater detail in the next chapter. It is important to review any material prior to using it in the classroom. You should look for material that is current and of high caliber. Some schools even make their own videos utilizing faculty and students. You also need to ensure that any electronic equipment is in good working order and be prepared with a backup plan in case your technology does not work.

Simulation is now widely used in both theory and clinical courses. There is a wide array of simulation equipment and resources that range from the simple to the complex. Simulation is a wonderful way to offer students hands-on experiences in a safe and controlled environment. Developing a simulation entails a lot of planning and there are specific guidelines on how to prepare, run, and evaluate a simulated experience. They can be done with mannequins or live actors and at times are video recorded so that students can learn from their mistakes by watching their own performance. If your academic setting does not have a simulation lab you may want to do role playing in the classroom. Role playing is a great way to get students to be active learners and most students enjoy this activity. A role playing experience should be well planned and specific roles and directions should be given to all participants.

A guest speaker who is an expert on a topic is another great teaching strategy and many professionals will come on a voluntary basis or for a small stipend. Always check with administration about the policy for guest speakers. It is a good idea to request a resume or CV so that you can review their qualifications. To arrange for a guest speaker you will need to plan in advance and be sure to discuss the specific content that he/she will be teaching. You will need to arrange for parking, hand-outs, and audio-visual equipment. Because most organizations are trying to be environmentally friendly, course material is often made available via a course management system to cut down on paper use and costs.

Self-learning modules with review questions and writing assignments may also be utilized to teach some of the content. You should carefully consider which content is best taught with this method. In general complex topics should not be taught via this method.

Creating a rubric (see Exhibit 8.3) for grading writing assignments is highly recommended because grading papers is subjective. Game playing can also be a fun way to learn and is often used for reviews with question and answers. Games can be done in teams or individual with token rewards. If carefully planned and used intermittently throughout the semester games can be a wonderful way to support and reinforce knowledge. These types of assignments help students to be independent learners and develop critical thinking skills (Billings & Halstead, 2009).

These are some common teaching strategies but there are others you may want to use and it is fun to be creative and think about new and different types of teaching and learning activities. Just be sure they are related to your course objectives and learning outcomes and are based on the evidence. If you are trying something new, you can evaluate its effectiveness through student feedback and formal evaluations.

Clinical teaching is somewhat different and you will be guided by the philosophy of your school and your own personal philosophy along with the expectations of the curriculum that is guided by accrediting and licensing agencies. According to Gaberson and Oermann (2010) "The competent role of the teacher in the clinical setting is competent guidance. The teacher guides, supports, stimulates, and facilitates learning" (p. 2). Gaberson and Oermann (2010) identified the following expected outcomes in a clinical course:

- Knowledge acquisition
- Ability to problem solve
- Development critical thinking
- Ability to make decisions
- Developing psychomotor skills
- Developing interpersonal skills
- Organizational skills
- Attitudes and values (caring, safety, quality)
- Cultural competence

EXHIBIT 8.3

Grading Rubric Template

Criteria	Level 1 Poor	Level 2 Fair	Level 3 Good	Level 4 Exemplary	Score	Comments
Content	Content is incomplete	Some points are addressed	Major points are addressed	All points are addressed and supported		
Organization	Poorly organized	Some organization	Good introduction and use of headings and conclusion	Paper flows well from introduction to conclusion		
References	Outdated and inadequate	Some current references	Several current references	All references are current and relevant from peer reviewed journals		
APA Grammar Spelling	Multiple errors	Several errors	Few errors	No errors in APA, spelling, or grammar		

Name: _____

Topic: _____

Grade: _____

Date: _____

Teaching and learning strategies in clinical include guided discussions during pre- and post-conference role modeling, simulations, observation, completion of skills checklists, individual instruction, written assignments such as care plans, concept mapping, journals, process recordings, and reflective papers, and summative and formative evaluations. Developing an individualized teaching and learning plan for each student is recommended. Clinical experiences should be related to the course objectives and learning outcomes and all assignments should be aimed at a specific learning outcome. Although many clinicals are pass/fail clinical faculty must evaluate students' performance and should keep weekly anecdotal records. Students should be given a copy of the evaluation tool that will be used for their formative and summative evaluations so they know what is expected of them. They may also be asked to complete a self-assessment that can be shared during the formative and summative evaluation meetings. The formative evaluation is usually completed midway through the semester and the summative is done at the end of the semester. However, if there are any concerns with performance or behavior, a conference should be held before the formal evaluation meeting. Be sure to follow proper protocol for notifying course coordinators and/or the dean about any students who are at risk of failing or are deemed unsafe in the clinical setting. There are many opportunities for teaching and learning in the clinical setting. Being organized and having a plan will help to ensure that all students have a positive learning experience and meet all the learning objectives and learning outcomes of the course.

SUMMARY

This chapter was on course planning and creating course syllabi, goals, objectives, and learning outcomes. Several teaching and learning strategies were reviewed for both theory and clinical courses.

DISCUSSION QUESTIONS

1. List the key components of a course syllabus.
2. Compare and contrast goals, objectives, and learning outcomes.
3. Compare and contrast the original and new versions of Bloom's taxonomy.
4. Identify the main differences in the cognitive, affective, and psychomotor domains.
5. Describe teaching strategies that were discussed in this chapter and how you would use them.

SUGGESTED LEARNING ACTIVITIES

▨ Utilizing the template, develop a course syllabus for a topic in your field of expertise.

▨ Develop a course offering utilizing the template at the end of this chapter.

▨ Identify and develop at least one or two teaching and learning strategies to teach your course.

REFERENCES

Anderson, L. W., & Krathwohl, D. R. (Eds.). (2001). *Taxonomy for learning, teaching and assessing: A revision of Bloom's Taxonomy of educational objectives: Complete edition.* New York, NY: Longman.

Bastable, S. (2003). Nurse As Educator: Principles of Teaching and Learning for Nursing Practice. New York: Jones and Bartlett

Billings, D. M., & Halstead, J. A. (2009). *Teaching in nursing: A guide for faculty* (3rd ed.). Philadelphia, PA: W.B. Saunders.

Bloom, B. S. (1956). Taxonomy of *educational objectives*, Handbook I: *The cognitive domain.* New York, NY: David McKay Co Inc.

Eber, P. A., & Parker, T. S. (2007). Assessing student learning: Applying Bloom's taxonomy. *Human Service Education, 27*(1), 45–53.

Gaberson, K. & Oermann, M. (2010) *Clinical teaching strategies in nursing* (3rd ed.). New York, NY: Springer Publishing Company.

Hermann, J. (2008) *Creative teaching strategies for the nurse educator.* Philadelphia, PA: FA Davis.

Thompson, B. (2007). The syllabus as a communication document: Constructing and presenting the syllabus. *Communication Education, 56*(1), 54–71. doi: 10.1080/03634520601011575

UNCC (2011). *Writing objectives using Bloom's taxonomy.* Retrieved from lesson plan rubric—for writing objectives using Bloom's taxonomy teaching.uncc. edu/.../GoalsAndObjectives/BloomWritingObjectives

University of Connecticut. (2011). *How to write program goals.* Retrieved from assessment.uconn.edu/docs/HowToWriteObjectivesOutcomes.pdf

Wolfe, K. (2004). Course materials–Syllabus and textbooks. *Journal of Teaching in Travel & Tourism, 4*(4), 55–60. doi: 10.1300/J172v04n04.05

ADDITIONAL READING

Mavrikos-Adamou, T. (2008). Syllabus construction: Designing an effective syllabus. *Conference Papers—American Political Science Association—Teaching & Learning,* 1.

CHAPTER 9

Technology and Course Management Systems

"We cannot teach people anything; we can only help them discover it within themselves."

— GALILEO GALILEI

OBJECTIVES

After reading this chapter, the reader will be able to
- Identify key components of a course management system
- Develop a PowerPoint presentation
- Discuss various technological pedagogies
- Compare and contrast online and hybrid courses
- Discuss advantages and disadvantages of using simulation

INTRODUCTION

This chapter will focus on technology and its application and use in higher education. This is an exciting time to be an educator because there are so many new advances in technology and with each passing year technology becomes more innovative and user friendly. Course management systems are used by many colleges and universities and offer the educator a wide variety of options in course facilitation. Use of technology in the classroom and how to develop a simulation scenario will also be discussed. An overview of online and hybrid/blended courses will also be presented.

COURSE MANAGEMENT SYSTEMS

A course management system such as ANGEL, Blackboard, or Moodle has become an essential part of most academic settings especially in higher education. Course managements systems are web-based computer programs that teachers use to manage their courses. Each faculty member has an account where all courses currently being taught are given an individual site. Faculty utilize these systems to communicate and share information with students. Course rosters are available with individual student email addresses. Course content can be uploaded and accessed by all students enrolled in the course. Some of the features include: course rosters and attendance logs, grade books, discussion boards, areas to upload content and course syllabi and outlines, email capabilities, and drop boxes for assignments. Students enroll in courses they are registered for and have access under student privileges and can view only their own information. A course management system enables you to run your course effectively and efficiently. You can access it from your home or office and it is relatively easy to navigate and there are always experts from the Information Technology Department who can support you while you're learning the system. Each course management system is unique but most of them share similar capabilities. The course management system is an integral part of your course and saves time and paper and reduces printing costs. Faculty can upload PowerPoints and other documents for their students to view before or during class. Many students have laptops so instead of printing tons of documents they can view them online. You can also include links to the library and other resources. Another great feature is the discussion board. This is a great way to create an interactive teaching session. You can post one or two questions related to the readings and have students respond throughout the week. Or you can post case studies and concept maps to be completed. Discussion boards are a wonderful way to help students develop critical reasoning and thinking skills and to stay connected between formal in-class meetings. The grade book enables you to post individual student grades while maintaining confidentiality. You can set up your grade book with all the required tests and assignments with the allocated percentage points so students know exactly how they are doing and how they are progressing throughout the semester. Of course, it is still a good idea to keep a hard copy of your grade book as a back-up. Another great feature is to use the drop box for assignments or as an attachment to an email. You can grade the paper as a Word document and insert comments and edits with the track changes function available in Microsoft Word. Then you can save the edited and graded paper and send it back to the student. It is a great way to manage written assignments and you always have a record of the student's work. Course management systems are of great value and will continue to be upgraded and offer many services to help faculty and students throughout their academic journey (Lawrence, 2006; Goyal & Purohit, 2009).

ELECTRONIC GRADING PROGRAMS

Grading exams can be a lengthy and laborious task but the use of an electronic grading system such Scantron can make the task much more efficient. There are many types of systems with different features and hopefully your academic setting will have one available for grading exams. Students need to bubble their answers on a special answer sheet and then these sheets are graded via the Scantron machine that is connected to a computer and printer. Results may include test grades, item analysis, reliability scores, and individual and group reports. The information is very helpful in analyzing your exams and also for establishing reliability and validity of test items. If your exam contains essays of short answers, you will have to grades those separately. Use of a rubric for grading essays is highly recommended.

TECHNOLOGY IN THE CLASSROOM

Today most classrooms are equipped with some type of technology that is used by a majority of teachers. Audiovisual equipment is the most common with PowerPoint presentations being the most popular. Some classrooms are already equipped with necessary equipment but at times faculty will have to request AV equipment. The use of PowerPoint presentations involves several things. First you should make sure that the computer/laptop, projector, speakers, and screen are available and are in good working order. Then you need to develop your PowerPoint presentation. You may already have this program installed on your computer or can purchase it for a fee. PowerPoint is relatively easy to use and a great tool for creating your presentations. It is important to develop high-quality, error-free presentations. PowerPoint presentations should have bullets of information with limited words (see Exhibit 9.1). They say a picture paints a thousand words so using clip art and other graphics is recommended. (Paradi, 2011) Other points to consider are background, font size and color, and layout. PowerPoints can be animated and also have sound added to them. Students can print up "hand-outs" or "note taking" versions of your presentation to help them take notes during class. This helps to cut down on student writing and allows them to pay attention to the presentation.

EXHIBIT 9.1

Examples of PowerPoint Slides

PowerPoint Slide 1 (Recommended)	PowerPoint Slide 2 (Avoid)
Leadership Style • What is your leadership style? • What type of leadership do you prefer?	Theories on leadership date back to the 19th century. There are many types of leaders. Some believe "leaders are born" and others believe "leaders are made." Leadership style can be autocratic, democratic, or laissez fairer. Some people make good leaders and others do not. Attending a leadership development course can be helpful.

The PowerPoint should be used to supplement your presentation and should contain the key points that you are going to discuss in greater detail. There are many wonderful resources online that you can review when developing your own PowerPoint presentations.

High quality DVDs and CD ROMS may also be used to supplement lessons but should be previewed first and used sparingly throughout the lecture. Students can view many of these in the learning center or library and would prefer to be taught by you instead of the video. There are some programs in nursing that have virtual hospitals and are interactive and can be used for group learning (Exhibit 9.2). They usually involve a patient scenario and students must click on the appropriate choice in the care of the patient. With each decision a different patient outcome is achieved. These programs facilitate critical thinking and help to relate theoretical concepts to the clinical care of patients.

Some classrooms are equipped with interactive white boards (Smart Boards) that look like a big white screen but have computer capabilities and enable you to highlight, type, and make your presentation more interactive.

EXHIBIT 9.2

Simulation Scenario-Sample

This scenario is based on a 55-year-old male patient who was recently experienced rectal bleeding and was diagnosed with Colon cancer Stage II and is one day post-op from a colon resection and colostomy. His vital signs have been stable.

The patient is going through the stages of grief and is in the anger stage. His wife and daughter are grieving. His wife is having a hard time accepting the fact that her husband has a colostomy. His daughter is afraid that he is going to die and miss her wedding.

During this scenario the patient is receiving the incorrect IV fluids and is complaining of pain but was just medicated two hours ago. Also the patient has an order for demerol but he is allergic and has an allergy band on his wrist. He also is going into CHF because he did not have his Inderal or Lasix yesterday and was also receiving excessive fluids.

The patient has a history of mitral valve stenosis and is on Inderal 20 mg po BID.

His post-op medication orders include: Clear liquids advance to regular diet as tolerated.

Incentive Spirometer q1h
Nasal O$_2$ at 3 l pm
Ceftriaxone 1.5 g q12h

Inderal 20 mg PO BID
Demerol 50 mg IM prn for pain
Percocet 2 tabs prn for pain
Ringer's lactate at 75 cc/hr

He is allergic to penicillin and demerol.
He is on a clear liquid diet.
He has a left transverse colostomy. Dressing dry and intact with colostomy bag. Bowel sounds are present but there is liquid brown stool in the colostomy bag.
He has a Foley catheter in place with 50 mL of clear yellow urine.
IV Normal saline at 125 mL/hr.
Lower extremities are edematous +2
Lungs have bibasilar rales.
In part one of this scenario the expected learning objectives and performance of the nurse:

To Complete Post-op Care of the Colostomy Patient
Conduct a patient assessment
Identify abnormal assessment findings (decreased urine output, breakthrough pain)
Pain management
Contact MD for pain management
Identify incorrect type and amount of IV solution
Safe medication administration
Develop a plan of care
Direct the nursing assistant to change the colostomy bag
RN must assess the stoma
Patient teaching (post-op care, use of incentive spirometer)

In the second part of the scenario the expected learning objectives and performance of the nurse are to:

Identify fluid and electrolyte imbalances
Think critically
Assess and identify a patient in respiratory distress
Lungs-Bibasilar rales.
BP 140/90, HR 110, RR 24 T-99.6
This includes assessment of respiratory rate, O_2 sat, edema, rales
Laboratory data (H and H normal, sodium-150, K-6.0)
Contact MD for respiratory management

(continued)

Roles will include a nurse and a nurse's aide, the patient's wife and daughter, and two observers.

The patient will be angry but not refusing care.

The nurse should be completing interventions based on the assessment findings.

Nurse needs to know what she can delegate.

Nurse's aide will be trying to do more than she should and tells the family members to leave.

Family will be wife and daughter . . . Wife can't look at husband and daughter is crying.

The observers will record findings every one to two minutes.

Debriefing will take place with group after simulation scenario.

QUESTIONS

For the nurse:

How did you feel during this experience?
What did you learn?
What would you have done the same or different?

For the nurse's aide:

How did you feel being told what to do?
What would you do if you did not agree with the nurse?

For family members:

What did it feel like to be in this situation?
Did the nurse and nurse's aide treat you how you expected to be treated?
Did you feel they provided safe and effective quality of care?

Some faculty use podcasting as a supplement. The presentation or lecture is recorded and then students can upload it to an I-Pod or MP3 player.

Podcasting has many applications in the educational setting and is especially embraced by the Millenial generation who expect and require stimulating education. Podcasting can be used locally, nationally, and even globally to enhance learning. However, it does take a considerable amount of time and preparation to develop a presentation and faculty must prepare scripts that are interesting and then recorded using a special software program that must be uploaded so that students can download it onto their personal devices. Students, especially ones who are auditory learners can benefit greatly from this type of technology (Long & Edwards, 2010). Furthermore, Long and Edwards (2010) posit: "Podcasting can be used for students who are absent and miss on-campus sessions, to help them catch up on the missed instruction" (p. 99).

Podcasting is an emerging technology that should be considered by nurse educators as a way to supplement their course offerings.

The use of PDAs has become popular and students may use them in theory and clinical settings. A PDA is a hand-held computer device that gives students instant access to information about medications and disease processes among other things. Some schools make these mandatory for students and for others it is optional. The PDA offers students a compact way to access current information and should be considered when planning your programs. Some software companies will give the student a free PDA if they purchase their software. (George & Davidson, 2005)

The use of webcams has also become popular and enables students to interact with other students from around the globe. For example, a group of students can be in a traditional classroom and have a webcam set up and students in different locations can sign onto the account and participate in the discussion. It can even be used for students who need to be absent but still want to participate.

Wiki spaces are used to develop private discussion boards for a particular group of students. There are many free sites or larger sites which require a minimal fee. Faculty post discussion questions and students respond. All of the posts are visible and students can choose which posts they want to respond to. To identify different uses participants use different color fonts. The space is password protected so only invited guests can view and participate. This type of pedagogy promotes critical thinking and independent learning.

There are multiple programs and new and exciting technologies emerging all the time and as an educator you need to keep current and up to date on new educational technologies. It is important to investigate, research, and evaluate new technologies as they are introduced.

DISTANCE LEARNING AND VIRTUAL CLASSROOMS

The use of online education is an innovative pedagogy that has grown in popularity over the past decade. Many schools offer some type of online learning. An online class is created using a computer, the internet, and course management system. It has advantages and disadvantages. Classes may be 100% online or offered as hybrid or blended courses. Courses that are taught totally online do not offer any face-to-face instruction and students must be very disciplined because they work independently. In an online course the faculty serves more as a facilitator and guides the class through a series of learning activities such as weekly readings, discussion questions, and written assignments. Streaming videos may also be utilized. Faculty and students need to be proficient in computer technology and have an IT department that can support them throughout the course. Development and teaching of an online course is a complex process and is actually more time intensive than teaching a traditional class (Tallent-Runnels, Cooper, Lan, Thomas, & Busby, 2005; Wallace, 2003). Baran, Correira, and Thompson (2011) posit: "It is through the integration of technology into the pedagogical inquiry that teachers can go through a transformative process of examining the pedagogical potential of online technologies and constructing online learning experiences within their content areas" (p. 433). A course syllabus and outline are utilized and often e-books are utilized. All classes must be carefully planned in accordance with course objectives and outcomes.

Anderson (2010) concluded the following:

> Developing an *online* course is not just reusing an old syllabus; it requires developing content, instructions, activities, multimedia learning objects, and assessment rubrics appropriate for a dynamic, interactive learning environment. Content updates keep material current and meaningful. Students quickly spot dated information or learning activities or errors; *teaching* is more enjoyable when content and activities are fresh. Monitoring and participating in discussions, assessing students' work, and addressing questions (including technical questions) require dedication. (para. 6)

Faculty interested in teaching an online course should be aware of the time commitment and preparation required to facilitate a high-quality course. Taking an online class is a good way to gain experience before teaching your own course. Starting with developing and teaching a hybrid/blended course is a way to "test the waters" to discover if online teaching is something you will enjoy. Many academic settings offer their faculty a certification course on how to teach an online course to better prepare them for this type of pedagogy. Utilizing the discussion board in your course management system or on a wiki space is a good way to experience one of the components of online teaching. Online courses are usually asynchronous so faculty and students have a lot of flexibility and can participate at whatever time of day works best. In hybrid/blended courses there is a mix of face to face and online classes. An example of a hybrid/blended model is 60% face to face and 40% online. Hybrid courses offer structure yet some level of flexibility. Some students prefer this method because they get the "best of both worlds" and enjoy the personal connection with faculty and other students. In general many adult students prefer online courses because it offers them more flexibility and they can also attend courses in virtually any location. Not all students enjoy online courses and some may hesitate because they do not know what to expect but teaching an online course can be a very rewarding experience.

VIRTUAL PROGRAMS

Another program that has become popular but somewhat controversial in educational circles is Second Life(SL), which is a virtual program that includes the use of an avatar and an ability to interact with other avatars. SL is a popular virtual program that is used for recreation and education. It is an online virtual world where individuals select avatars to navigate through the different worlds and locations. (Inman, Wright, & Hartman, 2010). Many schools now have virtual classrooms and libraries that are used for instruction and group work. "SL represents the most mature of the social virtual world platforms, and the high usage figures compared with other competing platforms reflects this dominance within the educational world" (Warburton, 2009, p. 416). SL is used by many educators to supplement learning. It offers a wide variety of uses and works well in groups and enables students to interact with other students and faculty from different parts of the world (Skiba, 2007).

According to Skiba (2009)

> Higher education is using SL to recruit and retain students, to teach classes, and as supplementary learning experiences. SL is all about experiential learning, being immersed in a virtual environment. It adds another dimension to simulations and allows for role playing, collaboration, real-time interactions between students and faculty, and experimentation. (p. 129)

Although the use of programs such as SL have become increasingly popular, additional research is warranted into this unique pedagogy. It is certainly something to consider, especially in nursing education.

SIMULATION

Simulation has been used for many years in education by a variety of disciplines. In recent years simulation has become increasingly popular especially in the field of nursing education (*Blum, Borglund, & Parcells, 2010*). Because of advances in technology the mannequins of yesteryear have advanced into computerized and interactive high-fidelity manikins that have heart sounds, lung sounds, and even body fluids. Simulation labs mirror real-life hospital rooms and with a little bit of imagination one can feel like they are caring for a real patient. Although many simulations are done with high-tech or low-tech mannequins there are some that are even done with live actors and actresses. Sometimes simulations are taped and students can view and critique them at a later date. Similar to every other pedagogy simulations have advantages and disadvantages and require extensive planning and coordination. Sanford (2010) identified advantages such as being able to create scenarios in a safe environment, and as a substitution for clinical hours because it is increasingly challenging to find clinical sites. However, only some states allow simulation to be counted as clinical experience so it is important to verify this with your state education department before using this in place of onsite clinical experiences. Disadvantages include lack of research and evidence, and length of time it requires for instructors to develop, set up, and run a simulation. Clearly there is a need for additional research and while some faculty are not enthusiastic about simulation there are proponents.

According to Jeffries (2009):

> A few states now allow up to 25 percent of real clinical time to be accounted for with the use of simulation. Jeffries predicts that as more

evidence is produced and best practices are developed, the use of the high fidelity simulators as well as much higher tech simulators will occur. (as cited in Sanford, 2010, p. 1010)

In support of simulation, Cant and Cooper (2010) conducted a review of the literature on the use of high-fidelity mannequins and concluded that simulation was an effective method for teaching and learning in nursing. However, they did note that further research is warranted in this area to develop a universal method for measuring outcomes. Although further research is warranted the use of simulation in nursing education is widely used and many educators are eager to utilize and conduct research in the area of simulations. Students also enjoy learning through simulation as they are able to practice in an independent yet safe environment. This type of pedagogy is especially helpful for kinesthetic learners who learn best with hands-on experiences. There are many resources that faculty can utilize to develop high-quality scenarios that meet the specific objectives and outcomes of their courses. The key to a successful simulation is preparation and facilitation. The use of simulation will continue to expand and with continued research should prove to be a highly successful teaching and learning strategy (Brewer, 2011).

SUMMARY

This chapter focused on technology and its application in nursing education. An overview of various pedagogies was presented in the areas of simulation and online education. The use of a course management system was also reviewed in addition to several other technologies that are currently being utilized. Although technology has been widely embraced further research needs to be conducted to determine the efficacy of these innovative teaching and learning methodologies.

DISCUSSION QUESTIONS

1. List the major components of a course management system.
2. Discuss three areas of technology and how you would use them in the classroom.
3. Compare and contrast the differences in an online and hybrid/blended classroom.
4. Discuss advantages of the online classroom.
5. Compare and contrast the advantages and disadvantages of using simulation in nurse education.

SUGGESTED LEARNING ACTIVITIES

▪ Develop a PowerPoint presentation on a topic of your choice.
▪ Create a wiki space for discussion of a topic from this chapter.
▪ Conduct a literature search on the use of online education in nursing and develop a course syllabus for a hybrid course.

REFERENCES

Anderson, M. (2010). What's it like to teach an online class? *Multimedia & Internet@Schools, 17*(6), 20.

Baran, E., Correia, A., & Thompson, A. (2011). Transforming online teaching practice: Critical analysis of the literature on the roles and competencies of online teachers. *Distance Education, 32*(3), 421–439. doi: 10.1080/01587919.2011. 610293.

Blum, C., Borglund, S., & Parcells, D. (2010). High-fidelity nursing simulation: Impact on student self-confidence and clinical competence. *International Journal of Nursing Education Scholarship, 7*(1), Article 18. doi: 10.2202/1548-923X.2035.

Brewer, E. P. (2011). Successful techniques for using human patient simulation in nursing education. *Journal of Nursing Scholarship, 43*(3), 311–317. doi: 10.1111/j.1547-5069.2011.01405.x.

Cant, R. P., & Cooper, S. J. (2010). Simulation-based learning in nurse education: Systematic review. *Journal of Advanced Nursing, 66*(1), 3–15. doi: 10.1111/j.1365-2648.2009.05240.x.

George, L., & Davidson, L. (2005). PDA use in nursing education: Prepared for today, poised for tomorrow. *OJNI, 9*(2) [Online]. Retrieved from http://ojni.org /9_2/george.htm

Goyal, E., & Purohit, S. (2009). Study of Using Learning Management System in a Management Course. *SIES Journal Of Management, 6*(2), 11-20.

Inman, C., Wright, V. H., & Hartman, J. A. (2010). Use of second life in K-12 and higher education: A review of research. *Journal of Interactive Online Learning, 9*(1), 44–63.

Jeffries, P. R. (2009). Dreams for the future of clinical simulation. *Nursing Education Perspectives, 30*(2), 71.

Lawrence, D. H. (2006). Blackboard on a Shoestring: Tying Courses to Sources. *Journal of Library Administration, 45*(1/2), 245–265. doi:10.1300/J111v45n0114.

Long, S., & Edwards, P. (2010). Podcasting making waves in millennial education. *Journal for Nurses in Staff Development, 26*(3), 96–101.

Paradi, D. (2011). *How to avoid "Death by PowerPoint" solving the five most common problems with powerpoint presentations.* Retrieved from www. thinkoutsidetheslide.com/articles/avoid_death_by_ppt.htm

Sanford, P. G. (2010). Simulation in nursing education: A review of the research. *The Qualitative Report, 15*(4), 1006–1011. Retrieved from http://www.nova. edu/ssss/QR/QR15-4/sanford.pdf

Skiba, D. J. (2009). Nursing education 2.0: A second look at second life. *Nursing Education Perspectives, 30*(2), 129–131.

Skiba, D. J. (2007). What is second life and nursing education. *Nursing Education Perspectives, 28*(3), 156–157.

Tallent-Runnels, M. K., Cooper, S., Lan, W. Y., Thomas, J. A., & Busby, C. (2005). How to teach online: What the research says. *Distance Learning, 2*(1), 21–27.

Wallace, R. M. (2003). Online learning in higher education: A review of research on interactions among teachers and students. *Education, Communication & Information, 3*(2), 241.

Warburton, S. (2009). Second life in higher education: Assessing the potential for and the barriers to deploying virtual worlds in learning and teaching. *British Journal of Educational Technology, 40*(3), 414–426. doi: 10.1111 /j.1467-8535.2009.00952.xW.

ADDITIONAL READING

Moodle (2012, April 25). About Moodle. Moodle.org: open-source community-based tools for learning Retrieved from moodle.org

Unal, Z., & Unal, A. (2011). Evaluating and Comparing the Usability of Web-Based Course Management Systems. *Journal Of Information Technology Education*, 1019–38.

CHAPTER 10

Evaluation of Learning

"You cannot open a book without learning something."
    —CONFUCIUS

OBJECTIVES

After reading this chapter, the reader be able to
- Discuss test development and construction
- Understand Bloom's Taxonomy
- Identify types of test questions
- Understand importance of item analysis
- Identify alternative forms of evaluation
- Discuss process of clinical evaluations

INTRODUCTION

Today more than ever a culture of assessment is at the forefront of education. Experts and educators alike recognize the importance of assessing everything from student learning, courses, teachers, and programs. The quest for sound assessment and evaluation methods is one that is challenging and requires creative thinking and formal testing of these methods. Often times methods are utilized that have not been adequately researched. Although many educators are participating in formal studies to identify evidence-based best practices, there is still more work to be done.

Evaluation and assessment of what has been learned are equally as important as what you have taught. Assessment is an ongoing process; Earl and Giles (2011) point out that assessment serves many purposes and is used to evaluate student learning and teaching abilities. Assessment includes both formative and summative information. The formative is the assessment that occurs throughout the course and the summative takes place at the end of the course. This enables both teachers and students to measure progress and develop plans to enhance learning and motivation to learn. The summative evaluation details if and how well the student achieved the expected learning outcomes. There are many ways to evaluate learning and most faculty use a variety of methods such as formal testing, written work, homework, observation, completion of formative and summative evaluations, checklists, and self-evaluation. When developing evaluation methods one must consider a student's learning style and past experiences. Not everyone is a good test taker and at best exams give you only a snapshot at that particular moment in time. Exams are also difficult to create and may not really measure expected learning outcomes. Many external factors such as stress, exhaustion, and fatigue affect a student's ability to do well on an exam. Evaluating students in the form of written work may be helpful. However, many students, especially if they were not educated in this country, may find writing particularly challenging. There are a number of ways you can evaluate learning through assessment and testing and an overview of these will be presented in this chapter. It is important to note that this is just an overview. Most graduate programs for nurse educators include an entire course on assessment, measurement, and evaluation of teaching and learning. There are also many wonderful resources available for new and experienced nurse educators that should be reviewed on a continual basis.

ASSESSMENT AND EVALUATION

Assessment and evaluation are related but different concepts. Bastable (2003) posits: "The process of *assessment* is to gather, summarize, interpret, and use data to decide a direction for action. The process of *evaluation* is to gather, summarize, interpret, and use data to determine the extent to which the action was successful" (p. 494). Therefore, faculty must select tools and methods to assess and evaluate student learning and program objectives in relation to their course goals, objectives, outcomes, and methods of instruction. Faculty must also perform a self-evaluation and are subject to evaluation by students, peers, and administrators, as well as program outcomes. Furthermore, continued evaluation and assessments are also conducted on programs, courses, clinical sites, and curriculums. The results of these assessments are utilized to improve courses, curriculum, and individual teaching.

Evaluation is an integral part of the teaching and learning process and educators use a variety of methods to evaluate student progress, knowledge development, and achievement of expected learning outcomes. Developing evaluation methods can be quite challenging and it is important to utilize more than one form of evaluation. It is also vital to use evaluations that are based on the evidence and that have been analyzed for validity and reliability. Validity is the ability of the evaluation or assessment method to capture the appropriate data. There are three main types of validity, which includes content related, criterion related, and construct related. Content related looks at whether the instrument measures expected outcomes; criterion related compares two different instruments; while construct related compares results of instrument to other scores such as IQ. Reliability is when a test or instrument that is used yields consistent results. Interrater reliability can be obtained by having two different teachers grade the same assignment using a rubric and then comparing scores to a measured agreement between scores. Test–retest is usually not a good method to use in exams because you would have to administer the same test to the same group of students and they would most likely do better. Using a split halves method for reliability may work better for exams (Billings & Halstead, 2009). It is important to evaluate whatever methods you employ to assess learning.

There are two main ways that evaluation can be done:

1. Norm-referenced assessment (NRA), according to which students are compared against each other as in ranking or grades; that is, A, B, C, etc. but these grades are unable to identify whether learners have achieved the goals set in the objectives of the program. NRA results are expressed after the teaching is over.

2. Criterion-referenced assessment (CRA), in which performance is evaluated at regular intervals during the course and results show progress towards criteria set in the curriculum. NRA makes judgment about individuals; CRA makes judgment about performance (Biggs 2003, as cited in Fardows, 2011, p. 35).

When planning a course you must decide what evaluation methods you are going to utilize before you begin your course. As previously discussed, some schools may have standardized or required exams and tools that must be utilized by all faculty. Students should know the types of evaluation methods that will be used and the due dates for submission of all assignments. Building in testing dates in your weekly course outline is also a great way to stay organized and help students plan for exams and projects.

BLOOM'S TAXONOMY

The original six domains in Bloom's Taxonomy are knowledge, comprehension, application, analysis, synthesis, and evaluation (Bloom, Englelhart, Furst, Hill, & Krathwohl, 1954). The updated domains which were reviewed in the previous chapter are remembering, understanding, applying, analyzing, evaluating, and creating (Anderson, 1994; Bloom, Engelhart, Furst, Hill, & Krathwohl, 1956). Many testing and evaluation methods are developed based on this taxonomy which increases in level of complexity. Many educators, especially in the discipline of nursing, utilize Bloom's Taxonomy to guide the development of testing and evaluation methods. For example, the National Council of State Board of Nursing has utilized both the original and updated versions of the taxonomy to develop NCLEX test questions that are mainly at the application or higher level in order to evaluate knowledge, skills, application, problem-solving, complex thought processing, and cognitive ability (National Council of State Boards of Nursing [NCSBN], 2010). In undergraduate nursing programs faculty develop tests utilizing the taxonomy and select domains based on course level. In lower-level nursing courses faculty may develop test questions based on knowledge/remembering and comprehension/understanding. As students progress to the higher and more complex levels, faculty develop higher-order questions such as in the domains of application/applying and analysis/analyzing. The highest levels are synthesis and evaluating. Many faculty develop tests that utilize several cognitive and behavioral domains so that they can measure different objectives. Creating methods of assessment and evaluation and test development and construction is very challenging and using taxonomy is just one part of this very complex task.

ASSESSMENT AND EVALUATION METHODS

There are many strategies faculty develop and utilize to measure effectiveness of teaching and learning strategies, cognitive development, knowledge acquisition, behavioral development, problem-solving ability, and critical reasoning skills. These methods include, but are not limited to:

- Formal testing with the use of various methods of examination
- Writing assignments
- Homework
- Participation
- Standardized tests
- Group projects
- Evaluation of psychomotor skills with return demonstrations and skills checklists
- Observation
- Completion of formative and summative evaluation tools
- Self-evaluation

As stated previously, faculty must decide which assessment, testing, and evaluation methods they are going to utilize during course preparation. It is best to use several different methods. One must also consider the type of course being taught and the expected outcomes.

The evaluation and assessment methods used should be aimed at assessing student learning and be based on the course goals, objectives, and learning outcomes. Each method should correlate to the syllabus and should reflect the specific outcome to be measured (Iran-Nejad & Stewart, 2010). Methods chosen should relate to the cognitive, affective, or psychomotor domains in one of the levels of Bloom's Taxonomy. Thus you may use role play and demonstration to evaluate psychomotor skills, or a writing assignment for cognitive or affective domains, or a portfolio for high-level cognitive domains and for formative and summative evaluations (Billings & Halstead, 2009). In an online course environment, assessment and evaluation may differ slightly, but may effectively be achieved through degree of course participation, quality of discussion question responses, and evaluation of written assignments using a predetermined rubric for grading. In a theory course, assessment and evaluation may be achieved with quizzes, exams, and written assignments with the most weight being allocated to the exams. In a clinical course, assessment and evaluation are achieved with formative and summative evaluations, observation, and completion of skills checklists. New faculty members will need mentoring and support in this area; it is expected that new faculty will seek guidance and help from mentors and experienced faculty members.

TYPES OF EVALUATION METHODS

Many undergraduate faculty utilize tests and quizzes to evaluate learning, especially in nursing programs. Tests can be used to measure cognitive and affective domains and to evaluate lower-order and higher-order thinking and learning. Exams may be criterion referenced, which measure individual performance, or norm referenced, which measure student performance in comparison to other groups of students. These comparison groups may be part of the class or part of a larger group of students (Oermann & Gaberson, 2009).

Exams

A popular type of measurement in undergraduate nursing programs is an oral or written exam. Most faculty develop their own exams either individually or as a group. These exams are comprised of different types of questions. The most common type of question in nursing is multiple choice. This option likely reflects the educators' desire to prepare students for the NCLEX-RN© exam, which uses a variety of multiple-choice types of questions. In general, utilizing a good selection of question types is recommended as it allows for evaluation in relation to individual learning style and expected learning outcomes. Each test item must be given a weight and most often the weight is equal for all test questions (Oermann & Gaberson, 2009). However, with essay questions a higher weight is allocated. There are some limitations noted with the use of multiple-choice questions and evaluating higher-level thinking. For example, Wendt and Kenny (2009) posit:

> Although there is agreement that item development at the application and analysis level is essential for the measurement of critical thinking, there appears to be increased evidence of the use of higher order thinking when examinees answer constructed response items requiring that the answer be written or typed. (p. 150)

Wendt and Kenny (2009) found that there are theoretical and empirical studies that support the efficacy of *constructed-response* items to evaluate higher-order learning. These types of questions require a written or typed response from the test taker. Wendt and Kenny (2009) completed a study on entry level nurses and the use of alternative testing items and found that the participants believed that the alternative questions were more difficult but more realistic than multiple-choice questions.

Examples of alternative test questions are short answer, fill-ins, essays, case studies, matching columns, and true/false questions. Creating a blue-print or test plan is highly recommended. You want to decide what topics will be included and how many questions will be included per topic. You will also need to decide the level of questioning. Depending on the course and placement in the curriculum some exams questions may all be at the highest level or you may decide to use a different level of questioning throughout the exam based on complexity of material. Another consideration is the length of the test and how much time you will allocate for completion. Many faculty give students a study guide or test plan to help them study. There are two schools of thought on this and you will need to do some research and make an informed decision on whether to post a study guide for your students.

Developing Multiple-Choice Questions

Developing reliable and valid questions takes time and practice. All multiple-choice questions are developed with three parts. The *stem* is the main part and may be in the form of a statement or a question. The stem should be written with positive statements instead of negative ones. It is best to avoid words like *no* or *not* and if you are going to use the word *except* it should be bolded or underlined. The *answer* section is usually comprised of four choices with one correct and best answer or in a multiple-response some or all of the choices may be correct. The answer choices should make sense and be written in a manner where the answer does not "jump right out at you." Furthermore, the choices should be similar in length and make sense. The *distracters* are answer choices that are plausible yet incorrect. They should also be similar in length to the other choices and be plausible. The distracter may also be correct but just not the best answer (Campbell, 2011).

Many textbooks come with programs that generate tests. You can use these programs to develop tests utilizing the test generator and the test bank questions or you can just use the test generator to create a test with your own questions. It is best to develop your own questions and just utilize the test generator program to format your exam. If possible always have an experi-enced faculty member review and critique your exam. Tarant and Ware (2008) point out that many multiple-choice questions are written poorly. Examples of poorly written questions include: ones with words such as *never, always, not,* and *except*; ending a stem with *a* or *an* may unwittingly give clues to answers; answer choices of all the above or none of the above; and stems that are unclear or grammatically incorrect. A study was undertaken by Tarrant and Ware (2008) to evaluate the effect of poorly developed exams on student achievement. The researchers found that lower-achieving students do better on poorly written tests and that many faculty still create exams using words that should be avoided such as absolute and negative words. Clearly there is a need for faculty to be better prepared in the development of high-quality exams.

Other Types of Questions

Short-answer questions can be written as questions or statements. These questions work well when you are assessing knowledge or recall of information. They should be clearly written with specific directions for completion. Be clear with directions and you will need to decide before the exam what answers you will accept.

Essays are another way to assess knowledge and critical thinking skills. There are many ways to utilize essays. For example, you can list a scenario and have students analyze or evaluate. Or you can have students write a compare and contrast essay on two similar disorders.

Students can be asked to critique or develop or explain a particular issue. Be sure to allow students enough time to complete their essays and also enough space to write their essays. It is also a good idea to develop a clear set of guidelines and a rubric so you can be more objective when grading an essay. An example of an essay question is as follows: compare and contrast two different yet similar diagnoses such as hyperthyroidism and hypothyroidism. Directions would include for students to discuss and then compare and contrast risks, etiology, manifestations, diagnostic tests, collaborative care, nursing diagnosis and interventions, medications, and patient education. This would be rather extensive so would be weighted more heavily.

True/false questions may be utilized when assessing knowledge and recall and comprehension. Questions are formulated with statements about a particular topic. The statements should make sense and be written in a way that makes the students think about the answer choices.

Matching questions are another good way to test knowledge and ability to recall. In a matching question there are two columns: one with statements or questions, and one with answer choices. There are usually four to eight questions matching questions. They should be similar in length and used for a specific learning objective (Conderman, 2002).

TEST BLUEPRINT

It is helpful to map out a test blueprint for each exam you create. The test blueprint identifies the number and weight of questions to be included in a test. An example of a test blueprint for endocrine disorders is as follows:

Pathophysiology	10 questions = 20 (2 points each)
Diabetes	10 questions = 20 (2 points each)
Thyroid Disorders	10 questions = 20 (2 points each)
Addison's and Cushing's	10 questions = 20 (2 points each)
Essay	= 20 points
Total Points	100 points

Questions will include 35 multiple choice, 1 matching column (worth 4 points), and 3 short-answer style questions.

PORTFOLIO ASSESSMENT

The use of portfolios in higher-order teaching and learning is well documented in the literature. Some educators are also using portfolios for assessment and evaluation. Baeten, Dochy, and Stryuven (2008) investigated the use of portfolios and assessment with a group of 138 first-year undergraduate business students. Contrary to their belief, the results of this study did not demonstrate a positive relationship between use of portfolio assessment and deeper approach to learning and higher grades. Furthermore, the researchers concluded that students preferred formal and standardized testing. If this method is going to be used, students will need to understand the benefits of portfolio assessment. This type of assessment may be more applicable in higher level courses (McMullan, Endacott, Gray, Jasper, Miller, Scholes, & Webb, 2003).

GAMES AND CLICKERS

A different type of assessment involves the use of game playing and peer review for assessing and evaluating knowledge. Charlier and Clarebout (2009) investigated the use of games with a group of 28 students who were taking a first-aid course. Citing issues with traditional testing such as stress, anxiety, and poor test performance prompted the researchers to explore other options. Gaming has been used in teaching and learning and is generally considered interesting, fun, and motivating. However, assessment with gaming has been limited. The participants in the study were evaluated with a traditional written test and with a game-based assessment. The game-based assessment was developed with a board game format and peer evaluation. The researchers found that most students liked this method of testing and that their mean scores were significantly higher than the scores they earned on their written exams. Furthermore, even the students who did not like game playing scored well. This type of assessment definitely has merit but requires further investigation and a significant amount of preparation on the part of the faculty.

Adults learn best with active learning approaches. Clickers are a great way to achieve this type of teaching and learning. They stimulate active learning and help students to stay interested and engaged in the lesson. Clickers are electronic hand-held devices that enable students to respond to questions. The questions are uploaded into a PowerPoint type of presentation and then each individual student responds to the question via a clicker or automated response system. This method immediately demonstrates, using a bar graph, how students responded to the question. It gives each student an equal opportunity to participate and can serve to stimulate discussion on the topic. Meedzan and Fisher (2009) conducted a study on this type of teaching and learning tool with a sample of 28 sophomore nursing students. They utilized the seven principles of good nursing education (Chickering and Gamson, 1991) to guide the development of their study. The principles include: interaction between the teacher and student; student-student interaction; active learning; time on task; rich, rapid feedback; communicates high expectations of the student's ability to learn; respect for different talents; and ways of learning. Meedzan and Fisher (2009) found that students had a high level of satisfaction with this type of technology and recommend continued research and faculty development on the use of this innovative technology.

Scoring and Grading

Scoring and grading are additional responsibilities of faculty. Exams must be scored to reflect the number of correct and incorrect responses and then graded based on weight of each item and the number of correct responses. When exam scores are lower than expected, some faculty, after analysis of all items may decide to drop some questions or curve overall grades. Before doing this, you should check the policies of the school and consult with senior faculty and/or administration. You must also follow a specific format for curving a grade and it must apply to all students' grades. Developing a sound and well-written exam may help to avoid having to make a decision about curving grades. The caveat to all decisions is to be fair and employ one standard for all students.

ITEM ANALYSIS

Determining how well a test has measured the desired learning outcomes is an important component in the assessment and evaluation process. Most academic settings utilize a computer-generated grading system that also has software that can generate reports with item analysis, discriminate analysis, and correlation coefficients. There are also formulas that can be done with paper and pencil to analyze the effectiveness of your exam. Whether using a computer or analysis by hand you must understand the statistical terms and what they mean in the evaluation of your exam. There are a number of ways you can evaluate test items but the important thing is do the analysis and use those results to improve your exam. Hamzah and Abdullah (2011) describe a process of analysis for evaluating an exam. First, exams are graded and divided into three main categories; high, average, and low. Next, a measure of central tendency is obtained by measuring the mean, mode, and median of the scores. Then, a discriminative index analysis (item analysis) is obtained for each item. An item is considered to have high discriminative index if the higher-achieving students answer it correctly and the lower-achieving students answer it incorrectly. This is the result you hope to achieve for a well constructed test item.

Hamzah and Abdullah (2011) state:

> However, if these two groups are able to answer the same questions correctly, the value of discrimination is zero. Also, if the less intelligent students answer a same question more than the more intelligent students, the value of discrimination is negative. These two situations are the ones we wish to avoid for a text item. (p. 315)

Finally, the difficulty percentage analysis is completed by counting the percent of students who answered the question correctly. Items should be moderately difficult with 50–80% of the students getting them correct. This also helps to establish reliability of the test items. In multiple-choice questions the distracter should also be analyzed. A distracter is considered valid if students who choose the incorrect choice choose the distracter. On the other hand, if most students choose the correct answer, then the question is most likely too easy. It is important to review each exam and use the information to improve future exams.

CLINICAL EVALUATION METHODS

A clinical course requires a very different type of assessment and evaluation than a theory course. The goal of the clinical experience is for students to develop knowledge, skills, and attitudes that will prepare them for professional practice. "Nursing as a practice discipline, requires development of development of higher level cognitive skills, values, and psychomotor skills for care of patients across settings" (Oermann & Gaberson, 2009, p. 245). Because of the complexity of the healthcare system and the ever-changing profession of nursing it is difficult to evaluate clinical competence. Furthermore, because most of the assessment and evaluation are achieved through observation by the clinical faculty the results are based on subjective findings (Walsh, Bailey, & Koren, 2009). Faculty most often utilize a tool that has been developed and approved by all the faculty in accordance with philosophy, theoretical framework, accrediting, licensure, regulatory standards, course objectives, learning outcomes, and curriculum of the school. A skills checklist may also be utilized to evaluate student competence in completing clinical skills and assessing psychomotor abilities. Some schools also use formal testing and assign letter grades instead of pass/fail grades. Assessment is ongoing and faculty provide feedback on a weekly basis regarding progress and achievement of expected outcomes. Feedback should include constructive information. Students should be told what they are doing well and where they need to improve. A formative evaluation is completed mid-semester and involves observation and assessment and feedback to the student. Throughout the formative assessment students should have an opportunity to develop a plan for improvement and to participate in experiences that will help them to develop and meet the expected outcomes. The summative is completed at the end of the semester. The summative evaluation is a compilation of the formative evaluation and determines if the student has met all the expected objectives and outcomes to pass the course. Written assignments may be required in the form of care plans, concept maps, reflection, journals, process recordings, and scholarly papers. To address the issue of subjectivity and evaluation some faculty are now using objective structure clinical evaluation (OSCE). Because of the limited research and evidence in relation to this method, Walsh et al. (2009) completed an integrative review. They reviewed 23 studies that had been conducted on the use of this type of evaluation. The OSCE involves simulation that entails students rotating through various simulated experiences and completing certain tasks.

Each station is constructed to assess a particular skill such as history taking, physical assessment, identifying a diagnosis, decision-making, client education or the performance of a technical procedure. The skills performed are assessed against a pre-established detailed checklist developed by a panel of clinical/education experts (p. 1586).

The researchers concluded that a gap in the literature remains on the evaluation of psychometric properties of this type of evaluation and warrants further research. This seems to be true of many of the current assessment and evaluations methods currently employed in education. Because clinical instruction is integral to the professional practice of nursing new methods of evaluation should be continually developed and tested in order to reflect current practice.

SUMMARY

This chapter discussed assessment, testing, and evaluation. Methods of assessment, and evaluation in addition to various types of questions were also included. The importance of developing well written exams and statistical analysis of results was reviewed. The process for clinical evaluation was also discussed.

DISCUSSION QUESTIONS

1. Compare and contrast the difference between assessment, evaluation, and testing.
2. Discuss methods of assessment and evaluation.
3. List and describe three different types of test questions.
4. Compare and contrast formative and summative evaluations.
5. Discuss ways to analyze a test using statistical measures.

SUGGESTED LEARNING ACTIVITIES

▪ Develop a 20-question exam using Bloom's Taxonomy and at least three different types of questions.
▪ Develop a clinical evaluation tool for a clinical course of your choice (Foundations, Med-Surg, Peds, OB, Psych, Community, or Leadership).

REFERENCES

Anderson, L. W. (1994). Research on teaching and teacher education. In L.W. Anderson & L. A. Sosniak (Eds.), *Bloom's Taxonomy: A forty-year retrospective* (pp. 1–8). Chicago, IL: The University of Chicago Press.

Baeten, M., Dochy, F., & Struyven, K. (2008). Students' approaches to learning and assessment preferences in a portfolio-based learning environment. *Instructional Science, 36*(5/6), 359–374. doi:10.1007/s11251-008-9060-y.

Bastable, S. (2003). Nurse As Educator: Principles of Teaching and Learning for Nursing Practice. New York: Jones and Bartlett.

Biggs, J. B. (2003), Teaching for Quality Learning at University' 2nd ed. Buckingham: SRHE and Open University Press, United Kingdom.

Billings, D. M., & Halstead, J. A. (2009). *Teaching in nursing: A guide for faculty* (3rd ed.). Philadelphia, PA: W.B. Saunders.

Bloom, B. S. (1956). Taxonomy of educational objectives, Handbook I: The cognitive domain. New York, NY: David McKay Co Inc.

Bloom, B. S., Englelhart, M. D., Furst, E. J., Hill, W. H., & Krathwohl, D. R. (1954). *Taxonomy of educational objectives: The classification of educational goals. Handbook I: Cognitive Domain.* New York, NY: Longman.

Campbell, D. E. (2011). How to write good multiple-choice questions. *Journal of Paediatrics & Child Health, 47*(6), 322–325. doi:10.1111/j.1440-1754.2011. 02115.x.

Charlier, N., & Clarebout, G. (2009). Game-based assessment: Can games themselves act as assessment mechanisms? A case study. *Proceedings of The European Conference on Games Based Learning,* 404–411.

Chickering, A. W., & Gamson, Z. F. (1991). *Applying the seven principles for good practice in undergraduate education. New Directions for Teaching and Learning, no. 47.* San Francisco, CA: Jossey-Bass.

Conderman, G. (2002). Writing Test Questions Like a Pro. *Intervention in School & Clinic, 38*(2), 83.

Earl, K., & Giles, D. (2011). An-other look at assessment: Assessment in learning. *New Zealand Journal of Teachers' Work, 8*(1), 11–20.

Fardows, N. (2011). Investigating effects of evaluation and assessment on students learning outcomes at undergraduate level. *European Journal of Social Science, 23*(1), 34–40.

Hamzah, M., & Abdullah, S. (2011). Test item analysis: An educator professionalism approach. *US-China Education Review, 9*(3a), 307–322.

Iran-Nejad, A., & Stewart, W. (2010). Understanding as an educational objective: From seeking and playing with taxonomies to discovering and reflecting on revelations. *Research in The Schools, 17*(1), 64–76.

McMullan, M., Endacott, R., Gray, M., Jasper, M., Miller, C., Scholes, J., & Webb, C. (2003). Portfolios and assessment of competence: a review of the literature. *Journal of Advanced Nursing, 41*(3), 283–294. doi:10.1046/j.1365-2648.2003. 02528.x.

Meedzan, N., & Fisher, K. (2009). Clickers in nursing education: An active learning tool in the classroom. *Online Journal of Nursing Informatics (OJNI), 13*(2), 1–19. Retrieved from http://ojni.org/13_2/Meedzan_Fisher.pd

National Council of State Boards of Nursing. (2010). Report of findings from the 2009 LPN/VN practice analysis: Linking the NCLEX-PN® examination to practice. Chicago, IL: Author.

Oermann, M. H., & Gaberson, K. B. (2009). *Evaluation and testing in nursing education* (3rd ed.). New York, NY: Springer Publishing Company.

Tarrant, M., & Ware, J. (2008). Impact of item-writing flaws in multiple-choice questions on student achievement in high-stakes nursing assessments. *Medical Education, 42*(2), 198–206. doi: 10.1111/j.1365-2923.2007.02957.x.

Walsh, M., Bailey, P., & Koren, I. (2009). Objective structured clinical evaluation of clinical competence: an integrative review. *Journal of Advanced Nursing, 65*(8), 1584–1595. doi: 10.1111/j.1365-2648.2009.05054.x.

Wendt, A., & Kenny, L. E. (2009). Alternate item types: Continuing the quest for authentic testing. *Journal of Nursing Education, 48*(3), 150–156.

CHAPTER 11

Legal Issues for Nursing Faculty

"The time is always right to do what is right."
—Martin Luther King, Jr.

OBJECTIVES

After reading this chapter, the reader will be able to
- Discuss federal and state education laws
- Understand academic freedom
- Identify issues in academic integrity
- Discuss legal issues and nurse educators
- Compare and contrast academic and disciplinary procedures
- Discuss legal issues of faculty and students

INTRODUCTION

An important but sometimes misunderstood issue relates to the legal and ethical aspects of higher education. There are many statutes and regulations that faculty must understand. Legal issues are related to your role as a faculty member, your role as an educator, and your role in clinical practice. There are federal statutes, along with state laws and regulations in regards to admissions, re-admission, discrimination, disciplinary action, and dismissal from a program. Policies and procedures should be well written and strictly adhered to when addressing any of these aforementioned issues (Westrick, 2007). State boards of education develop and enforce many laws in regards to nursing education and faculty. Academic organizations consult legal counsel to help them to develop policies and procedures based on federal and state regulations. Faculty members need to be aware of all the legal and ethical issues that guide their practice and inform their role as educators in a practice discipline. In this chapter, an overview of the most common issues will be presented.

NURSE PRACTICE ACT

The Nurse Practice Act identifies the scope of practice for registered professional nurses. The National Council of State Boards of Nursing (NCSBN) has developed a model for individual states to adapt and amend based on the laws in their jurisdiction. Each state has its own state board that develops standards based on the national board and state laws. The following is the model that was developed by the NCSBN:

> **Practice of Nursing**. Nursing is a scientific process founded on a professional body of knowledge; it is a learned profession based on an understanding of the human condition across the lifespan and the relationship of a client with others and within the environment; and it is an art dedicated to caring for others. The practice of nursing means assisting clients to attain or maintain optimal health, implementing a strategy of care to accomplish defined goals within the context of a client centered health care plan and evaluating responses to nursing care and treatment. Nursing is a dynamic discipline that increasingly involves more sophisticated knowledge, technologies and client care activities. (NCSBN, 2005, p. 3)

All faculty and students must be knowledgeable about their individual state's Nurse Practice Act which informs and guides professional practice in the state. There are many rules and regulations that are established on a federal level and a state level in regards to education and licensure of nurses. Your academic organization will have specific policies and procedures in place to ensure compliance with all regulations and each individual teacher is also responsible for compliance. It is a good idea to visit the website of your particular state board of education so you can familiarize yourself with all of the related statutes and regulations.

FEDERAL LAWS PROTECTING RIGHTS OF FACULTY AND STUDENTS

Faculty and students are bound by the U.S. Constitution and the protection of rights such as the First Amendment on freedom of speech and the Fourteenth Amendment that includes the right to due process. Statutes on discrimination, privacy, and disabilities are also mandatory. These statutes apply to all public institutions and private institutions that receive federal funds. The Family Educational Rights and Privacy Act (FERPA) (20 U.S.C. § 1232g; 34 CFR Part 99) is a federal law that protects the privacy of student education records. The law applies to all schools that receive funds under an applicable program of the U.S. Department of Education (2012). It is important to note that students over 18 years of age have to provide written permission for their parents or legal guardians to view their records or discuss any other topic with faculty. The privacy of students must always be maintained and faculty must be cognizant of this when a parent calls to discuss any personal issue such as grades or performance. Unless the student has provided permission for faculty to discuss these issues with the parent or guardian, these types of discussions must be held with the student only and must be considered private and confidential. FERPA also dictates that grades must be posted in a secure manner.

Federal Acts That Govern Institutions Receiving Federal Funds

The following federal acts must be adhered to by any school, private or public, that receives federal funding:

▪ *The Age Discrimination Act of 1975* prohibits discrimination based on age in programs or activities that receive federal financial assistance, such as from the U.S.

DEPARTMENT OF EDUCATION
The Age Discrimination regulation describes conduct that violates the Act. The Age Discrimination regulation is enforced by the Office for Civil Rights and is in the Code of Federal Regulations at 34 CFR Part 110. OCR enforces two laws that prohibit discrimination based on disability.

▪ *Section 504 of the Rehabilitation Act of 1973* prohibits discrimination based on disability in programs or activities receiving federal financial assistance. The U.S. Department of Education gives grants of financial assistance to schools and colleges and to certain other entities, including vocational rehabilitation programs. The U.S. Department of Education's Section 504 regulation is enforced by OCR and is in the federal code of regulations at 34 CFR 104.
▪ *Title II of the Americans with Disabilities Act of 1990* prohibits discrimination based on disability in public entities. OCR is the agency designated by the U.S. Department of Justice to enforce the regulation under Title II with respect to public educational entities and public libraries. The Title II regulation is in the federal code of regulations at 28 CFR 35 Race and National Origin Discrimination (Title VI of the Civil Rights Act of 1964).
▪ *Title VI of the Civil Rights Act of 1964*, prohibits discrimination based on race, color, or national origin in programs or activities receiving federal financial assistance (U.S. Department of Education, 2012).

Breaches of any of these statutes or complaints of educational malpractice or breach of contract may result in legal action against the faculty or school and may be reported to the Office of Civil Rights. Because of this, colleges and faculty must keep careful records of all student files and be aware of the laws that govern education.

PROTECTING ACADEMIC FREEDOM

Academic freedom is valued and revered by most educators but often not fully understood. It continues to be a controversial issue and is the subject of many discussions and debates. "The traditional justification for academic freedom refs to the social role academics play in the discovery and dissemination of truth" (Andreescu, 2009, p. 500). Faculty must be guided by legal, moral, and ethical principles when applying their rights to academic freedom.

The American Academy of University of Professors issued the following statement:

> **Statement of Principles on Academic Freedom (AAUP, 1940, 1970 rev)**
> Teachers are entitled to freedom in the classroom in discussing their subject, but they should be careful not to introduce into their teaching controversial matter which has no relation to their subject. Limitations of academic freedom because of religious or other aims of the institution should be clearly stated in writing at the time of the appointment.

All faculty have academic freedom but must use this freedom in a responsible manner. They do have the right to express their opinions and to teach their courses without censure as long as they do not impinge on contractual agreements or the rights of the students. Faculty has the right to evaluate and grade their students based on their objectives. For example, an administrator cannot tell a faculty member to give a student a higher grade or change a grade. Faculty also has the right to pursue their own scientific inquiry and research. However, faculty does not have the freedom to change policies and procedures because they do not agree with a certain rule and regulations. There are many misconceptions regarding academic freedom and tenure. Some believe that tenured faculty can say and do whatever they want and cannot be fired. However, this is not accurate. Tenure does afford a faculty member a degree of security but does not excuse them from their roles and responsibilities. Also in the case of financial exigency by a college, tenured faculty may be lose their positions (Billings & Halstead, 2009). Some faculty feel that academic freedom is being taken away because of accrediting agencies and standardization of curriculum and courses.

Ledoux, Marshall, and McHenry (2010) posit:

> The implication is clear: accrediting agencies can deprive institutions, faculty, and students of academic freedom by attacking the individual's self-identity. Such pressure may presume to improve curriculum development and conceptual frameworks, but it can also harbor hidden personal and political agendas. (p. 252)

It is important to understand academic freedom and how it applies to your role as an educator. Being an educator is a very serious responsibility and it is important to use your freedom wisely. You also want to be sure that you protect your academic freedom for yourself and other educators. You can do this by staying informed and speaking out about infringements of faculty freedom. Faculty should be able to engage in research with a spirit of inquiry that will advance science and stimulate a further quest for knowledge.

LEGAL ISSUES AND FACULTY

Our country has become very litigious and you need to protect yourself and your organization from unnecessary lawsuits. Gunby (2008) posits, "In general, the courts have viewed faculty actions and decisions legally troublesome if the actions or decisions appear to be arbitrary, capricious, adversarial, or in bad faith" (p. 412). An example of this would be not following your own syllabus, the student handbook, or failing to follow the policies of the school. Having a detailed and clear syllabus and being sure to follow it will help to avoid many issues. Students must be treated fairly and equally. The student faculty relationship is reciprocal in nature and respectful. You want to develop a positive professional relationship with your students and be there to support them. It is important to begin and end class on time. If unforeseen circumstances cause you to cancel a class or be late for class, students should be notified as early as possible and a plan to make up the missed class should be developed. Students can sue a teacher and/or the academic organization for educational neglect if he/she does not fulfill the course requirements. There are also very specific laws regarding students with disabilities and faculty and schools must make reasonable accommodations for students. This will be discussed in greater detail in Chapter 19.

GRADING POLICIES

All policies must be adhered to for all students and should be established at the beginning of the course. If for some reason you do need to revise the syllabus you should seek guidance from administration and if approved you should have students sign an acknowledgment that they have received a copy of the revised syllabus. It is important to provide students with continuous feedback and to have formal meetings with documented plans for improvement during the semester. Grades are private and should be shared only with the student. Grades should never be posted with personal identifiers. If available it is best to post on your course management system. You should check with your academic setting as each school has different policies. Unfortunately, not every student will be successful but you want to do what you can to help them with tutoring, referrals, and support and be sure to keep a detailed record. You also want to be able to grade exams and papers in a timely fashion. Students should have their grades and feedback before their next test or assignment. This way they can use this information to identify areas for improvement. Some faculty have students sign learning contracts that clearly delineate the role of the faculty and the role of the student in the plan for academic success.

ADVISEMENT

Most faculty serve as advisors for an assigned group of students that they are responsible for in addition to the students they formally teach. As the advisor you are responsible for helping students navigate through their programs by selecting appropriate courses which include core courses, pre-requisites, co-requisites, course progression, and courses related to the particular major. Individual meetings are held throughout the semester to discuss progression, challenges and issues, and planning for the following semester. You also need to approve courses for students so they take the correct courses. Always be sure to document these sessions as per the policy of your school. A potential lawsuit would relate to the incorrect advisement of a student that resulted in them not being able to graduate or that delayed their graduation. You must be very familiar with the curriculum, including courses, prerequisites, co requisites, and placement in the program. It is helpful to develop your own system for advising students. You will be required to document electronically or in the student's personal folder. This is also a confidential meeting so be sure to maintain student's privacy. Whenever you are in doubt be sure to consult with someone regarding the issue. If you do make an error in advisement you must inform the student and other appropriate personnel and find a way to correct it.

Office hours are another responsibility of faculty and you must be available to meet with your students on a weekly basis for conferences and to discuss issues. Each academic organization has specific policies so always be sure to check. For example, you may be required to have 4 hours per week on at least two different days. Most faculty post their office hours on their course syllabi and outside their office doors. Unless an emergency arises you should be available to meet with students during your official hours or by appointment. If you need to cancel your hours, you should notify administration and find another time during the week to meet with students.

EDUCATIONAL MALPRACTICE

Faculty are responsible for keeping current with all new information, technology, policies and procedures, and teaching and learning strategies. Faculty must also be able to objectively assess and evaluate student outcomes. They must also be prepared and teach the required content. Although it is not possible to know everything, faculty must do their best to stay current and tell their students when they are unsure of something. Students will appreciate your honesty and everyone can go home and research it and discuss it at the next class. Any behavior by a teacher that negatively affects a student and/or the college may be identified as teacher misconduct. If students feel that there was a breach of contract in their educational process, they may accuse a teacher or an organization of educational malpractice. For example, if a teacher covers only 50% of the course content, students may feel they have not received the level of education they paid for when they registered. However, the student must prove that because of a breach of contract they were harmed or sustained some type of damage and this is often difficult to prove (McMahon, 2008; Scheetz, 2000).

> Educational malpractice is a tort cause of action. Essentially, a claim
> of educational malpractice asserts that educational institutions and

their employees breached their duty to educate plaintiffs adequately. Although educational malpractice has been the subject of much scholarly commentary (see, for example, DeMitchell & DeMitchell, 2003), it has been almost universally rejected by the judiciary. (Fossey, 2010, para 1)

Academic organizations may discipline or report faculty for various breaches of professional conduct which may be identified by students and teachers as potential areas for teacher misconduct. Nurse educators can utilize the National Education Association's Code of Ethics, the American Nurses Association's Code of Ethics, and the International Council of Nurses Code of Ethics to inform their practice (Sheetz, 2000). Furthermore, nurse educators should be well versed in ethics and moral judgments, inform their students on ethics, and be guided by the ethical principles of beneficence, nonmaleficence, autonomy, veracity, justice, fidelity, and confidentiality (Burkhardt & Nathaniel, 2002). McMahon (2008) found that both students and faculty identified the following areas of potential teacher misconduct: grade inflation, not addressing students' breaches of academic integrity, favoritism, giving or receiving expensive gifts, sexual advances, borrowing or giving money to a student, and inappropriate socializing with students. Faculty must be cognizant of all rules and responsibilities and maintain professional relationships at all times.

ACADEMIC INTEGRITY

Issues with academic integrity have become more prevalent in the past 20 years. Academic integrity has been defined as "a commitment, even in the face of adversity, to five fundamental values: honesty, trust, fairness, respect, and responsibility" (Center for Academic Integrity [CAI], 1999, p. 4, as cited in Tippitt et al., 2009). McCabe (2009) has been involved in an 18-year longitudinal nursing study on academic integrity and found that this issue has reached "epidemic proportions" (p. 614). Furthermore, at the onset of her study she thought that nursing students would have a higher level of integrity but unfortunately this was not the case, at least in her study. There are multiple integrity issues and some of the most common include: cheating on exams with cheat sheets, sharing answers, crib notes, electronic devices; copying; various types of plagiarism; not reporting clinical errors or documenting erroneous information; and taking credit for other students' work. The reasons students partake in academic dishonesty are varied and include a desire to succeed, fear of failing, not being prepared, and for the thrill of getting away with something (Sheetz, 2000). Faculty can help to prevent this by reviewing issues of academic integrity in their syllabi and during class. Students should also be aware of the possible sanctions, which include failing a test or written assignment, failing the course, and dismissal from the college. Faculty are responsible for maintaining standards and must address and report any issues of academic integrity. Failure to do so is a breach of academic integrity on the part of the faculty member. It is important to be a positive role model for students and serve as a highly ethical and moral teacher. You must set the tone and be clear in your expectations and be sure to be alert for any issues. Some schools use computer systems such as "turnitin" to identify any issues of plagiarism. Some schools use special testing rooms or have extra proctors in the room. Many schools have clear testing policies which may include: student identification, turning off electronic devices, nothing on desk except a pen or pencil, not being able to leave the room once testing has begun, no hats or scarves, calculators, pens and pencils provided by the teacher. There are many devices that students may use to cheat and faculty need to keep informed of these and other ways students partake in academic dishonesty. Students must also understand what constitutes a breach of academic integrity as they may not even realize that they have committed an academic violation. Students and faculty have a moral and ethical responsibility to report any violations that they observe. As a faculty member you must always base your decisions on facts and carefully follow all of the guidelines set forth by your academic setting. If time allows, always consult with your department chair or dean before formally addressing the issue to ensure proper protocol is being followed. It is important to clearly document the occurrence and have a formal meeting with the student to discuss the issue and consequences. A record of the incident should be placed in the student's file and you should also keep a copy for your personal records (Spain & Robles, 2011).

Students are also required to be punctual and attend classes and clinical on a regular basis. There are specific policies regarding this and in general absences are not allowed in the clinical area. Some schools allow for one emergency day that will have to be made up but more than one absence may result in a failure for a clinical course. This policy should be clearly communicated to students and as a faculty member you must keep careful records of attendance and punctuality. Students have the right to due process and may grieve or appeal a decision that they believe is fair or unjust.

LEGAL ISSUES AND CLINICAL STUDENTS

The clinical experience is fraught with potential issues of malpractice and unethical behavior. Faculty and students are responsible for providing high quality, safe, and effective patient care. Nursing students do not practice under the instructor's license as per the Nurse Practice Act: "Nursing students have the ultimate responsibility for their own actions and may be liable for their own negligence" (Wacker Guido, 2006, p. 505). The role of the clinical faculty brings an entire dimension of academic integrity. Patient safety is at the forefront of all clinical experiences and both faculty and staff are responsible for their own actions. Students should not be assigned to a clinical experience unless they have achieved the required level of competency required for the particular experience. However, faculty in the academic and clinical settings must set the standards and clearly communicate to the students what the expected behaviors and outcomes are for the rotation. Faculty must always be in attendance and be supervising students. Because they can observe only one student at a time faculty should be very clear in their directions to students in regards to which tasks may be completed independently and which ones must be supervised. Students are obligated to follow the rules and while faculty may bear some responsibility for the actions of their students the students are also responsible for doing what is expected. For example, students must understand that they may not administer medications without your direct supervision. A serious breach would be if the student administered the medication without your supervision. This would be grounds for a disciplinary action. Furthermore, if an error was made the student would bear the responsibility. And although you might be named in a lawsuit you would most likely be found innocent because your syllabus clearly stated that students were not allowed to administer meds and in doing so the student did not follow the policy (Scheetz, 2000). However, if as the instructor you assign patients who are too complex for the student or do not properly supervise the student, then you may be liable.

Another issue is with documentation in the medical record which is a very serious responsibility. The policies of the organization must be followed and students must clearly be identified as student nurse and documentation must be co-signed by the instructor/preceptor. Documentation must be accurate and confidentiality and privacy must be maintained. Falsifying records or failing to provide care for the patient is a serious legal and ethical issue. Another potential issue relates to errors in patient care, especially medication errors. Faculty and students must do everything in their power to prevent harm to patients by following all policies and procedures and carrying out assessments and prescribed orders in a timely and safe manner. If an error is made, it must be reported immediately so as not to cause further harm to the patient. Faculty and students should understand and follow the guidelines of the Joint Commission (National Patient Safety Goals, The Joint Commission [TJC], 2012) and also incorporate the six QSEN (Quality and Safety Education for Nurses) competencies. Both of these websites are listed at the end of this chapter for further review.

The six core competencies of QSEN are patient-centered care, teamwork and collaboration, safety, evidence-based practice, informatics and quality improvement (QSEN, 2011). These competencies were developed in an effort to address the serious and sometimes fatal errors that occur in the hospital. The rules of confidentiality and HIPAA must also be adhered to by faculty and students. While some breaches are of a malicious intent many are done inadvertently. For example, in the clinical setting patient information is highly confidential. Students and faculty should use only initials when discussing or when developing written assignments on specific patients. Medical records must not be copied or removed from the nursing unit. Charts should not be left out for others to view and computers are password protected. Patient information should not be discussed in public areas and must not be shared with anyone for any reason other than patient care. HIPAA violations can result in civil and legal lawsuits and fines.

SAFE ENVIRONMENTS

Providing a safe environment in which students can learn is a responsibility of the academic organization, the clinical organization, and the faculty. Students are vulnerable and must be protected from discrimination, sexual harassment, and all types of violence. There is a zero-tolerance policy for these types of behaviors. Faculty and students must be careful to avoid partaking in discrimination, sexual harassment, and physical or verbal abuse. These are serious issues that may result in disciplinary or legal action. There are times when faculty and students unwittingly offend someone so it is important to be respectful and to think about your words and actions. Workplace bullying affects all organizations and students are particularly at risk. Therefore, faculty must protect their students from being bullied and address any issues immediately. Faculty must also address and report issues of drugs, alcohol, or any criminal behavior. If the student is a danger to himself/herself or others, faculty must notify the appropriate authorities. The faculty has the right to send any student home who is not prepared for clinical or who poses a risk to patient safety.

The faculty/student relationship is extremely important, especially in the clinical setting and certain boundaries must be maintained. You are not there to be their friend, confidant, therapist, or win a popularity contest. You are there to teach and mentor your students in a caring and supportive manner. Because you are in a position of authority you must be careful not to abuse this role. You must develop a balance between instructing and constructive evaluation. There are times when you will need to counsel students on their behaviors and you want to do so in a professional manner. It is always good to try to acknowledge the positive behaviors along with the areas requiring improvement. Remember to always be respectful and conduct any evaluations or conferences in a private manner.

Faculty must help their students to understand safety issues in the clinical setting such as infection control, fire safety, and patient safety. Assignments should be fair and based on students' current level of competency. Faculty should guide their students and be sure to emphasize use of personal protection equipment and prevention of needle sticks. Faculty should always remind their students that while they should be respectful of the staff, they should take directions only from you as their instructor. If a staff nurse asks them to do something, they should know to check with you first. Most staff nurses want to help the students learn but they are not always cognizant of the competency level of the student or what the student is allowed to do without supervision. Of course each organization is unique and there are contracts between the school and the clinical agency that clearly delineate roles and responsibilities of all parties.

You must be aware of what your scope of practice is in your role as clinical instructor. Most clinical experiences are positive and following policies and procedures helps prevent negative experiences.

STUDENT RIGHTS, DUE PROCESS, AND GRIEVANCES

Students have the right to due process, fair treatment, confidentiality, and privacy (Billings & Halstead, 2009, p. 35). There will be times throughout your teaching profession that you may have to give students a negative evaluation, a failing grade, or a disciplinary action. All students have the right to due process and the ability to grieve a decision or appeal a grade. Guidelines for how to do this should exist, with each step clearly stated and should be readily available for students in the handbook. Faculty must follow the guidelines and complete any required actions and documentation for all infractions. Students are responsible for reviewing the guidelines and for filing their own grievances or appeals as per the policy. Wacker Guido (2006) described the differences between academic and disciplinary dismissal. An academic dismissal relates to the student's inability to successfully complete the required courses. All schools have specific grading policies and GPA requirements; students may be allowed to repeat one or two courses and still be retained in the program. When this happens students are usually placed on academic probation and have formal meetings with faculty, advisors, and deans. A plan for success should be developed and the student may be asked to sign a learning contract. If these measures are unsuccessful the student may be dismissed from the program. When this happens a meeting will be held with the student and other options will be discussed. Sometimes students can change their major and still remain in the school. Students can appeal this decision but must have reasonable cause such as breach of contract or unfair grading policies. Billings and Halstead (2009) describe procedural due process which is based on the Fourteenth Amendment and relates to the student's rights to be properly notified and granted a hearing. Substantive due process relates to the fact "that a decision must be fair, objective, and non-discriminatory" (p. 35). A disciplinary action or dismissal relates to infractions of rules, codes, or policies. Students must be provided with a written copy of the infraction along with the disciplinary measure. The students must also have an opportunity to defend themselves. All schools have a formal process for appeals which must be followed and careful records should be kept of every meeting. Initially there is a meeting with the faculty and the student; the next meeting may take place with the dean or the grievance committee. Students must be given an opportunity to defend themselves against the charge and may bring witnesses on their behalf. Depending on the issue it may be elevated to the provost or president of the college. Grievances do not involve formal legal representation at the hearing but legal counsel may be present to advise but not to question. However, after the hearing the student may consult with a lawyer and if the matter is not settled to the satisfaction of the student, he/she may decide to submit a formal lawsuit but that does not guarantee that the decision will be reversed. Faculty must abide by the decision of the appeals committee. It is important to have all records available to support the reason the student had an academic or disciplinary dismissal. You should retain course syllabi, tests, papers, anecdotal records, evaluations, and other applicable forms until a student has graduated. Students may also file a grade appeal if they believe they deserved a higher grade. However, if faculty has applied fair and objective practices in grading the grade will probably not be changed.

MALPRACTICE INSURANCE

All nurses should have their own malpractice insurance and as a faculty member, especially in the clinical setting, it is advisable to carry a higher amount. Although you will usually be covered under your school's plan, it is important to have your own coverage because you may be sued personally and not as part of your academic setting. Furthermore, as a clinical teacher, you may also be sued by a patient (Wacker Guido, 2006).

SUMMARY

This chapter provided an overview of legal issues in the academic setting. The issue of educational malpractice and how to avoid it was reviewed. Issues with academic integrity were discussed along with the importance of following the course syllabus and maintaining careful records.

DISCUSSION QUESTIONS

1. How do federal and state laws influence the role of nurse educators?
2. Discuss how academic freedom influences your role as an educator.
3. List five breaches of academic integrity and how you would address them. Include ways to prevent and address when they occur.
4. Describe the role of the educator in due process and student grievances.
5. Discuss ways you can prevent educational malpractice.

SUGGESTED LEARNING ACTIVITIES

- Read the following article and write an essay on your views of academic freedom:
  Krell, M. (2011). The ivory tower under siege: a constitutional basis for academic freedom. *George Mason University Civil Rights Law Journal*, *21*(2), 259–298.
- Interview a faculty member and a dean on academic freedom and compare and contrast their views.
- Conduct a review of the literature on issues of academic integrity and develop a lecture or PowerPoint presentation for students on the topic.

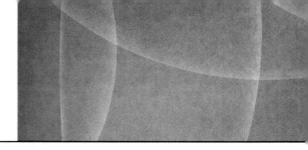

Curriculum and
Student Advisement

MARY ALICE HIGGINS DONIUS, EdD, RN

THE DEFINITION OF NURSING THAT GROUNDS the curriculum at The College of New Rochelle is that nursing is caring with compassion, empathy, and altruism with the intention of healing body, mind, and spirit. Often times when students fail to achieve course objectives or violate policy, they will plead to the faculty or dean to reverse the decision. One of the arguments students will make is to cite the definition and point out that the imposed sanction is "uncaring" and not reflective of our stated philosophy. This comment always gives pause for reflection. The question for me is not do we impose the necessary sanctions in order to maintain academic and performance standards but how do we do it in the context of a caring-healing curriculum. The definition of nursing offers guidance when preparing and conducting the disciplinary conversation with students.

The three concepts of caring: empathy, altruism, and compassion, can be used to frame the words and actions of the faculty member engaging in the conversation. *Empathy* is coming to know the other. Therefore, the faculty has to consider and appreciate the impact that the required decision will have on each student. Acknowledging the personal context will set the foundation for a caring interaction.

Altruism is actions taken to relieve the suffering of another. Imposing sanctions can seem the antithesis of an altruistic act. Faculty need to be aware of the presentation of potentially devastating information. The setting for the meeting, the words to be used, and the availability of support systems including time, tissues, and counseling need to be in place prior to the conversation with the student.

But perhaps the most important aspect of caring in these situations is to have a *compassionate* heart. Compassion is sharing the suffering of the other. Faculty may want to hurry the conversation because it is uncomfortable. But this is the time for making time. Making time to reflect on your own compassionate nature and how you will use your heartfelt connection with the student to avoid devaluing, dismissing, or disengaging with the student during the difficult conversation.

The ultimate key to the conversation as part of the disciplinary process is the intention of the faculty. Maintaining practice, professional, and institutional standards is the role of the faculty. The conscious awareness of your intention for the sanction as well the conversation in the context of healing body, mind, and spirit will help the student to hear the conversation in a different way.

The student's initial *body-physical* and *body-emotional* responses may be quiet, rational, or dramatic. Be prepared to deal with any and all responses by keeping focused on the objective nature of the discussion while acknowledging the appropriateness or inappropriateness of the response. Set the boundaries for safety and respect while supporting the student.

In the context of the mind, the goal is minimize the immediate personalization of being a failure. Keeping the focus on the specific failure or violation in the context of the action or outcome and not the personhood of the student will help the student come to an understanding and acceptance of the sanction. Statements such a "you are not a failure, you failed a course" or "you are not a bad person, you made a poor decision" may help students come to terms with what has occurred.

The aspect of *healing* is the most important to moving the student forward is addressing the concept of spirit. Faculty responsibility must include helping the student find meaning and purpose in what has happened. Students are not necessarily ready to engage in this dimension of the conversation. But the faculty needs to begin the conversation by providing a context for making sense of the event and considering the potential and possibilities the outcome of the event now provides. It may provide a deeper understanding of the course content and practice, a better respect for academic and institutional policies, or a more thoughtful consideration of professional and personal opportunities.

The *nurturing nature* of nursing faculty is readily acknowledged as an asset for helping students achieve academic success. When success is not possible, faculty may use their nurturing nature in the context of caring-healing to preserve the dignity of the individual and maintain the standards of the nursing profession and practice.

Tips for a Caring-Healing Disciplinary Conversation

Express *empathic* understanding
- Connect the behavior or outcome to the sanction
- Acknowledge the deep sense of loss

Utilize *altruistic* actions
- Be thoughtfully prepared by knowing the incident and the rules
- Prepare the space and outline the conversation

Keep a *compassionate* heart
- Be firm but gentle
- Reframe the event for acceptance

Set the *intention* for the highest good

Protect the *body-physical* and the *body-emotional*
- Respond with positive verbal and non-verbal statements while setting the limits
- Alert those whose assistance may be needed

Preserve the dignify of the *mind*
- Do not give false hope of reversal of decision
- Do not personalize to the student's core but to the sanction

Guide the *spirit* to find meaning and purpose
- Give hope by reframing the decision as an opportunity
- Continue to be a resource to the student

REFERENCES

Andreescu, L. (2009). Foundations of academic freedom: Making new sense of some aging arguments. *Studies in Philosophy & Education, 28*(6), 499–515. doi: 10.1007/s11217-009-9142-6

Billings, D. M., & Halstead, J. A. (2009). *Teaching in nursing: A guide for faculty* (3rd ed.). Philadelphia, PA: W.B. Saunders.

Burkhardt, M., & Nathaniel, A. (2002). *Ethics & issues in contemporary nursing* (2nd ed.). New York, NY: Delmar Thompson Learning.

Center for Academic Integrity (CAI) (1999). Retrieved from http://www.academicintegrity.org/icai/about-3.php.

DeMitchell, Todd A., & DeMitchell, Terri A. (2003). Statutes and standards: Has the door to educational malpractice been opened? *Brigham Young University of Education and Law Journal*, 2003, 485–518.

Fossey, R. (2010). Educational malpractice. *Education Law*. Retrieved from lawhighereducation.com/49-educational-malpractice.html

Gunby, S. (2008). Legal issues in teaching nursing. In B. K. Penn (Ed.), *Mastering the Teaching Role* (Chapter 31, pp. 411–421). Philadelphia, PA: F.A. Davis Company.

Ledoux, M. W., Marshall, T., & McHenry, N. (2010). The erosion of academic freedom. *Educational Horizons, 88*(4), 249–256.

McCabe, D. (2009). Academic dishonesty in nursing schools: an empirical investigation. *Journal of Nursing Education, 48*(11), 614–623. doi: 10.3928/01484834-20090716-07

McMahon, M. (2008). Teacher misconduct. *Teacher Misconduct—Research Starters Education*, 1–6.

National Council of State Boards of Nursing(2005). *Nursing Regulation and the Interpretation of Practice* retrieved from www.Nursing Regulation and the Interpretation of Nursing Scopes of ... https://www.ncsbn.org/NursingReg andInterpretationofSoP.pdf

National Educational Association. Retrieved from http://www.nea.org

QSEN. (2011). *Quality and safety education for nurses*. Retrieved from http://www.qsen.org

Scheetz, L. (2000). *Nursing faculty secrets*. Philadelphia, PA: Hanley & Belfus, Inc.

Spain, J., & Robles, M. (2011). Academic Integrity Policy: The Journey. *Business Communication Quarterly, 74*(2), 151–159. doi: 10.1177/1080569911404407

The Joint Commission (2012). National Patient Safety Goals retrieved from www. Accreditation, Health Care, Certification|Joint Commission www.joint commission.org/

Tippitt, M., Ard, N., Kline, J., Tilghman, J., Chamberlain, B., & Meagher, P. (2009). Creating environments that foster academic integrity. *Nursing Education Perspectives, 30*(4), 239–244.

Wacker Guido, G. (2006). *Legal And Ethical Issues In Nursing* (4th ed.). New York, NY: Prentice Hall.

Westrick, S. (2007). Legal challenges to academic decisions. *Journal of Nursing Law, 11*(2), 104–107.

U.S. Department of Education. (2012). *Civil rights*. Retrieved from http://www.ED.gov

ADDITIONAL READING

Hunt, Deborah (2012). QSEN Competencies: A Bridge to Practice Nursing Made Incredibly Easy!: September/October 2012 - Volume 10 - Issue 5 - p 1–3 doi: 10.1097/01.NME.0000418040.92006.70 Online exclusive

CHAPTER 12

Curriculum and Student Advisement

"Tell me and I forget. Teach me and I remember.
Involve me and I learn."

— BENJAMIN FRANKLIN

OBJECTIVES

After reading this chapter, the reader will be able to
- Identify key components of the curriculum
- Discuss theories that guide curriculum
- Understand the importance of curriculum and theoretical framework
- Understand the significance of NCLEX
- Discuss key issues in student advisement

INTRODUCTION

This chapter will focus on the relationship of nursing theory in the development of curriculum and programs. An overview of several theories will be presented along with the importance of academic advisement, the role of the advisor, and the licensure exam.

Nursing Theory

Since the days of Florence Nightingale and her concepts on the patient, nurse, and healing environment, the profession of nursing has been evolving. For many years nursing followed the medical model. However, nursing leaders knew that in order to be considered a professional discipline, nursing had to develop its own science that was based on scientific inquiry, research, and theory development. Walker and Avant (2005) posited: "Developing nursing's distinct knowledge base through theory development, research, and reflective practice was foundational to moving nursing from an occupation subservient to medicine to present-day partnership among the health professions" (p. 4).

There are four levels of theory in nursing: metatheories, grand theories, middle-range theories, and practice theories. The metaparadigm of person, nurse, health, and environment is the phenomena of concern to nursing educators, leaders, nurse researchers, and scientists. The four levels of theory can be depicted as a triangle with the metatheories on the top. Metatheory is broad and abstract and may include purpose, method, and criteria for testing theories in an attempt to explain the meaning of nursing as a science and a profession. They are the overarching theories that guide our research.

Grand theories are abstract and explain the broad purpose of the discipline and provide us with a perspective that is unique to nursing. Most of them were developed between 1960 and 1980. Examples of grand theories include Roger's (1970) "Humanistic Science of Nursing" and Watson's (1979) "Philosophy on Caring." Because grand theories are difficult to test, middle-range theories were developed. Middle-range theories are more concrete, with fewer variables and lend themselves to testing and evaluation. Examples of middle-range theories include "Comfort Theory" by Kolcaba (2001) and "Uncertainty Theory" by Mishell (1988, 1990). Practice theory is concrete and measurable. An example of a practice theory is Ruland and Moore's (1998) "Theory of the Peaceful End of Life" (Walker & Avant, 2005). "Dickoff and colleagues (1968) advocated a model of 'practice oriented theory' in which four phases of theorizing were to lead to the theory base for nursing practice. These phases included factor-isolating, factor-relating, situation-relating, and situation-producing or prescriptive theory" (Dickoff, James, & Wiedenbach, 1968a, as cited in Walker &Avant, 2005, p. 14). Nurse scientists utilize theories to guide both qualitative and quantitative research and inquiry to inform our practice and advance our science.

Theoretical Frameworks and Curriculum

The curriculum of a nursing program is informed by a conceptual or theoretical framework that relates to the mission and philosophy of the faculty and the mission of the school. Basically, it is a plan for preparing a nurse generalist through the development and leveling of all program objectives and outcomes, credit allocation, course content, and outcomes. Some programs espouse to one theory while other programs espouse to several theories that serve as the underpinnings or foundation of their curriculum. The curriculum belongs to the faculty and as such should reflect the integration of a sound theoretical base. The curriculum is also based on regulatory and accrediting agencies and program outcome goals. Concept and content mapping can be very helpful in planning the progression of a curriculum. Most schools have a curriculum committee that reviews, revises, and updates the curriculum and then presents it to the entire nursing faculty for approval.

As a faculty member, you want to be well versed in your program's philosophy and theoretical framework. Integration of theories should be evident in the program and individual courses. Required content is also threaded throughout the core courses. The curriculum must continually be updated to reflect the current standards and expectations of licensing and accrediting agencies and stakeholders. The central focus of the conceptual framework is the educational focus on nursing's metaparadigm of person, nurse, environment, and health.

Blaise, Hayes, Kozier, and Erb (2006) defined the metaparadigm as follows:

1. *Person or client*, the recipient of nursing care (includes individuals, families, groups, and communities)
2. *Environment*, the internal and external surroundings that affect the client, including people in the physical environment, such as families, friends, and significant others
3. *Health*, the degree of wellness or well-being that the client experiences
4. *Nursing*, the attributes, characteristics, and actions of the nurse providing care on behalf of or in conjunction with the client (p. 96).

Nursing programs share the common goal of preparing nurse generalists or advanced practice nurses. All nursing programs are most often accredited by one of the two major certifying bodies: the National League for Nursing Accrediting Commission (NLNAC) or the American Association of Colleges of Nurses (AACN). Some nursing programs are accredited by both. The conceptual and theoretical framework of nursing programs sets each apart from other programs. The American Association of Colleges of Nurses (AACN, 2008) recently has updated *The Essential of Baccalaureate Education for Professional Nursing Practice*. The *Essentials* document identifies standards for curriculum and outcomes of undergraduate and graduate nursing programs. For example, evidenced-based practice, genetics, geriatrics, holistic care, and QSEN recently have been added to the AACN *Essentials* document. Baccalaureate programs that wish to receive accreditation must address the *Essentials* in their curriculum. If you teach in a baccalaureate program or a master's program that is accredited by the Commission on Collegiate Nursing Education (CCNE) which is a subsidiary of the AACN, you should be familiar with the Essentials and accreditation standards which can be viewed on the AACN (2012) website. If you teach in a program that is accredited by the National League for Nursing Accrediting Commission (NLNAC), you will want to be familiar with the NLN accreditation standards which can be found on the NLN website. Both of these organizations offer current information and resources for nurse educators.

It is important to integrate and thread your philosophy and theoretical and conceptual framework throughout your program and individual courses. Students should also be knowledgeable about the theories that inform their program.

Nursing Theories and Curriculum

Nursing programs utilize a variety of different philosophies and theories to guide their curriculum. In this section, several often utilized philosophies and/ or theories will be highlighted to give a snapshot of some of the widely used concepts.

Martha Rogers (1970) developed the *Science of Unitary Human Beings Theory* and was instrumental in shaping nurse practice, education, and theory. Her theory has five basic assumptions:

1. human beings are whole beings who are more than the sum of their parts;
2. there is a constant changing of energy between the person and the environment;
3. life follows an irreversible pattern along the space and time continuum;
4. pattern and organizations identify whole individuals;
5. only human beings can have emotion, language, sensation, and abstract thinking (Alcantara, 2009; Rogers, 1989).

Henderson (1966) developed the *Need Theory* which has 14 components. It is credited with moving nursing away from the medical model by developing the following definition of nursing:

> The unique function of the nurse is to assist the individual, sick or well, in the performance of those activities contributing to health or its recovery (or to peaceful death) that he would perform unaided if he had the necessary strength, will or knowledge. And to do this in such a way as to help him gain independence as rapidly as possible. (Henderson, 1966, p. 15)

Hildegard Peplau (1952) developed the *Theory of Interpersonal Relations* which is considered a middle-range theory. This theory focuses on the nurse-patient relationship and included four phases; orientation, identification, exploitation, and resolution. According to Blaise et al. (2005), this theory continues to be used today, especially in mental health nursing.

Betty Neuman's (1982) *Systems Model* represents the client within the system perspective, wholistically and multi-dimensionally. It illustrates the components of five interacting client variables:

1. physiological
2. psychological
3. developmental
4. sociocultural
5. spiritual

These client variables act in relation to environmental influences upon the client as a system. These environment influences consist of basic structure, lines of resistance and lines of defense (Neuman, 2010).

Orem's (1971) Theory of Self-Care emphasizes four areas where individuals learn to care for themselves. The four basic components are self-care, self-care agency, self-care requisites, and therapeutic self-care demand (Taylor & Renpenning, 2011, p. 6).

Roy's (1976) Adaptation Model was developed by Sr. Calista Roy and has been widely used in nursing. In this theory there are five elements that include health, environment, nursing activities, goal of nursing, and person. The goal of nursing is to help patients develop adaptive behaviors. Behaviors are derived from regulator and cognator mechanisms and responses may be adaptive or ineffective (Nursing Theories, 2011, para. 22).

Jean Orlando (1961) developed the *Nursing Process Discipline Theory* that included assessment, diagnosis, planning, intervention, and evaluation. Her theory is a practice theory and focuses on the interaction between the nurse and the patient and the nursing process is widely used today in all aspects of nursing care.

Many programs embrace a caring philosophy and the theories of Jean Watson and Madeline Leininger. Although less well-known Blaise et al. (2005) identify Meyeroff (1971) as the "philosopher who provided much of the foundational work on the concept of caring" (p. 105). According to Watson (2009) many programs use her theory/philosophy to guide or change their programs both in the hospital and academic setting. Watson describes her theory in the following way:

> *This theory/philosophy involves making explicit human caring and relationship-centered caring is a foundational ethic for healing practices; it honors the unity of the whole human being, while also attending to creating a healing environment. Caring—healing modalities and nursing arts are reintegrated as essentials to ensure attention to quality of life, inner healing experiences, subjective meaning, and caring practices, which affect patient outcomes and system successes alike. This work places human-to—human-caring as central to professional nursing responsibilities, the role and moral foundation for the profession. Preserving human dignity, relationships and integrity through human caring are ultimately the measures by which patient's evaluate their often "cure dominated experiences.*
> (Watson, 2005, p. 51, as cited in Watson, 2009, pp. 470–471)

Schools of nursing may use Watson's theory by itself or with a combination of other theories that best meet the philosophy of their program. Many schools espouse a holistic caring/healing philosophy and holistic care is currently addressed in the *Essentials*. You can learn more about this theory by visiting Dr. Watson's website which contains a wealth of resources.

Leininger also worked on theories of caring; however, she also incorporated the dimension of culture in her *Theory of Culture Care: Diversity and Universality*. She is known as the founder of the transcultural nursing movement and coined the term "culturally congruent care." Her theory is widely used and embraced by many nurse educators. Leininger based her theory on anthropology and the work of Margaret Mead and thus helped nursing to realize that health and illness states are strongly influenced by culture.

Leininger describes her theory as being middle-range and believes that "caring is the essence of nursing." In Leininger's theory diversity addresses the unique health beliefs and practices of different cultures and universality as the commonalities of these beliefs among all cultures. Today, because of our very diverse society there has been a major emphasis on cultural competence and culturally congruent care (Leininger & McFarland, 2002).

Rosemarie Rizzo Parse (1992) developed the *Theory of Human Becoming.* One of the basic tenets of this theory is that the goal of nursing is to promote quality of life based on the patient's perspective. It includes the paradigms of simultaneity which states that man is a unitary being in continuous mutual interaction with the environment; and totality which states that man is a combination of biological, psychological, sociological, and spiritual factors. The three assumptions of this theory include meaning, rhythmicity, and transcendence.

Kolcaba developed her middle range *Theory of Comfort* in the 1990s. This theory identifies three of comfort: relief, ease, and transcendence. Kolcaba (1994) discussed the role of comfort in nursing and identified the need for conceptualization of the theory. Understanding her theory can positively influence holistic nursing care. "The theory of comfort provides direction for nursing practice and research because it entails an outcome that is measurable, holistic, positive, and nurse-sensitive" (Kolcaba, 1994, p. 1183).

Patricia Benner's model *Novice to Expert* has focused on the clinical development of nursing students and nurses and identifies five stages of development, which include:

1. novice
2. advanced beginner
3. competent
4. proficient
5. expert

A nursing student would be considered a novice and a new graduate nurse would be considered an advanced beginner (Benner, 1984).

Carper (1978) developed a framework on *ways of knowing* which included empirical knowing, aesthetic knowing, personal knowing, and ethical knowing. Empirical knowing is based on logical or positivist thinking and is based on evidence and quantitative methods. Aesthetic knowing relates to the "art" of nursing and caring and is based on qualitative and subjective findings. Ethical knowing relates to moral and ethical knowing and respect for human dignity.

Personal knowing relates to intuition and having an awareness of self and others. Recently, two new dimensions were added: unknowing and socio-political knowing. Unknowing relates to reflection and finding deeper meaning. Socio-political knowing relates to issues of nursing on a global level (Johns, 1995).

These descriptions provide an overview of some well-known theories and models but should not be considered an all-inclusive list. As a new nurse educator you should have a sound knowledge base of theories and models that guide the discipline of nursing. Importantly, you should have extensive knowledge of the theories and models that are used in your particular program.

Academic Advisement

Academic advisement is a serious responsibility of faculty and requires time and commitment and knowledge of your specific curriculum. The role of the advisor had been described as one that is highly influential. Furthermore, student satisfaction with their advisor has been linked to development of positive attitudes and experiences and retention. Students rely on their advisors to discuss issues such as personal values and specific information about their majors (Coll & Draves, 2009). Students rely on the faculty advisor to guide them throughout their program. They expect that the advisor will help them to select their required courses in the correct progression so that they can graduate when expected. Students and faculty both have responsibilities in this process but clearly the faculty member plays a more significant role. Students need to be guided throughout their academic journey and freshmen will need the most support and guidance as college is quite different than high school. Initial faculty advisement meetings with new students will focus on developing a working relationship and reviewing the overall curriculum, credits, and plans for the next four years. Many schools have forms they use that list the course progression and catalog descriptions that list the required courses and any pre- or co-requisites. One cannot assume that the student understands how to navigate all the nuances of college life. Many students do not understand how or why the curriculum follows a particular pattern and that they have to take courses in sequence. They are not always aware of pre-requisites or co-requisites. That is why most schools require mandatory meetings with faculty advisors and approval of courses prior to registration. In general students become more independent and confident as they progress in the program but are still required to have formal meetings. Registration is another component of advisement and students require an approval before they can register for a course. Course advisement and registration is just one component of the advisor's role, albeit a very crucial one. If students are not properly advised, they may not be successful or their graduation may be delayed. Students who are misadvised may sue the advisor or school for breach of contract.

Faculty also meet with their students to discuss issues such as academic challenges, failing grades, withdrawals, incomplete grades, and probationary status. Faculty advisors work with students to develop plans of success and strategies for studying and improving grades. Faculty may also inform students of the various support programs that may be available to them. However, students must also take responsibility for their success and you are not responsible if students do not follow your advice. That is why documentation of all interactions and meetings should be completed on all students. Many schools have a formal process for this which may be in an electronic form or in hard copy. It is important to have clear and concise notations about your student meetings and advisement. This way if an issue does arise you can show that you fulfilled your role. Furthermore, if you leave or become ill and another faculty member has to take over your student they will know exactly what occurred in the past. Most faculty are assigned a group of students for whom they will be the advisors for the semester, the year, or the entire duration of their program. Ideally you will have the same students from freshman year until graduation. This helps to develop positive relationships and you can advise students better when you know their specific strengths and weaknesses. You must schedule time for your advisees and meet according to the requirements of your school. For example, some schools require a formal meeting every quarter while others may require more frequent meetings. It is important to note that advisement is separate from office hours. Office hours are the time you are formally in your office to meet with any student from your classes, while advisement is time that is specifically set aside for you individual advisees. That is not to say that you cannot meet with an advisee during your office hours; it just means that you must allocate enough time to meet with all of your students. Students are responsible for making timely appointments with their advisor. As a new faculty member advisement can be daunting but if you are prepared and have a mentor you should do well. Sometimes, you are not required to advise during your first semester and will most likely have an opportunity to observe a senior faculty member during advisement. You may also have someone observe you initially and to be there as a support when you advise for the first time. You may also be given a lighter assignment so that you can learn at a slower pace. Your role as an advisor may also be considered when applying for promotion and tenure. With time and experience faculty advisement can be quite enjoyable and rewarding as you watch your group of students progress through the program. It is wonderful to see the learning and maturity that take place over a four-year period.

NCLEX

The National Council Licensure Exam (NCLEX) is taken by all graduate nurses in the United States to test their knowledge and skills at the completion of their programs. The major areas tested in NCLEX are safe and effective care environment, health promotion, psychosocial integrity, and physiological integrity. Schools of nursing prepare nurse generalists with the hope that they will be able to pass this exam and obtain their license. NCLEX pass rates are an important indicator related to program evaluation and a valuable program outcome. NCLEX pass rates are published on a quarterly and annual basis and are of interest to various stakeholders. Stakeholders include the students, communities, hospitals, and government. In addition to the formal curriculum and evaluation methods many schools use an NLCEX success program to help students to prepare for their licensure exam. As a faculty member you want to be sure that you are teaching content that is current and will help your students to begin their role as nurse generalists and be successful on their licensure exam. The NCLEX test plan is updated every three years to address new information, trends, and technology. You should review this information and also share it with your students. As a faculty member you can help your students prepare for their licensure exam by helping them to develop critical thinking and reasoning skills. Helping students develop test-taking skills especially in answering multiple-choice questions that are based on Bloom's Taxonomy for higher-order cognitive thinking will also be very helpful. Furthermore, you can teach students stress reduction techniques and strategies for pacing oneself and reading each question carefully. Administering practice exams on a computer will also help improve the student's ability to pass. Students need to become comfortable with answering computer-based questions that are timed and that do not allow the student to go back once the question is answered. Faculty should utilize their NCLEX pass rates to evaluate the effectiveness of their curriculum. If test scores are below level, then a plan for improvement should be developed. This plan should be based on a thorough assessment of all components of the curriculum followed by a comprehensive plan that has specific objectives and measurable outcomes for improving test scores. National Council of State Boards of Nursing (NCSBN, 2012).

SUMMARY

This chapter discussed the relationship of theory and nursing curriculums. An overview of a select group of conceptual and theoretical frameworks was presented. The role of student advisement was also discussed and the significance of NCLEX as a program outcome.

DISCUSSION QUESTIONS

1. How does theory inform the curriculum?
2. What are the four domains of nursing's metaparadigm?
3. Compare and contrast metatheory, grand theory, middle-range theory, and practice theory.
4. Discuss the faculty role as an advisor.
5. Discuss several ways you can help students pass their licensure exam.

SUGGESTED LEARNING ACTIVITIES

▪ Participate in different role-playing scenarios related to student advisement.
Suggested scenarios:
  – Freshman student
  – Failing student
  – Transfer student
  – Advisement error
▪ Select three nursing theorists and write a report on their theory and their contributions to nursing practice and education.
▪ Develop a plan for NCLEX success in a school that has a low pass rate.

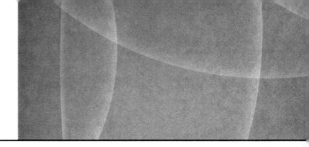

Teaching and Sustaining Human Caring

JEAN WATSON, PhD, RN, AHN-BC, FAAN

WELL, FIRST THINGS FIRST AND first things are the students, not the faculty, not you, not the content, nor the factual technical material that you assume as the teacher-expert.

It is first, students, and secondly you, being prepared. Be prepared to reach the students, honor the students, seek to get into their heart and mind with learning, not just content and facts, but knowledge and insights that are personally meaningful. Help them to gain confidence in themselves and make sense of their situation, their life and nursing context—to feel safe to learn.

A good educator is not content-driven, but driven by love, by passion, intellect, moral ideas, by your desire to inspire students to reach the highest level of their potential, even when they cannot see or believe in themselves. A good educator has a passion for scholarship related to human experiences and caring—healing—relationships—whether they be through human connections or technological connections, always sustaining the whole human context.

Nursing education is an act of love and caring. It is love of humanity, love of nursing, love of learning, love of diversity, love of challenge of ideas, love of knowledge, and love of sharing knowledge with kindness and patience, in ways that inspire, invite, and create safe space to listen, to ask questions, to disagree, and to evolve together. Be open to hear what students (and patients) have to teach you. You as *the faculty*, become the *expert learner* along with your students.

Personal teaching recall:

One of my first teaching experiences that stands out, was in the mid -1970s, with 120 students, in the first-year undergraduate nursing course, open to all nursing and psychology students:

"Psychological Growth and Development Across the Life Span." The topic for the week was psychological theories of growth and development of persons who were gay or homosexual.

I was approaching the class content, open and flexible, (as I thought I was—with my new PhD in social/educational/clinical psychology background, and my master's in psychiatric mental health nursing), via a conventional psychodynamic point of reference as one primary view in the psychological literature at that time.

The students did not agree with the psychodynamic, more conventional psychological theoretical developmental views; they wanted other diverse, contemporary social points of view to be incorporated to expand the discussion. The students asked to meet with me after the class and expressed their disagreements. I listened and honored their concerns.

Within a matter of minutes, after active listening and safe dialogue, we had created an open panel discussion for the next class. This included: a gay student, the parent of a gay man who was popular in the community (speaking from a parent's experience and perception), another student who was straight but had gay friends, another member of a gay organization in the community, along with several other panel members. It was a most exciting, socially current, relevant, and dynamic next class, which was co-created by the students and me in open and safe dialogue.

Students were safe to be critical, but also pro-active for new learning and personal insights into the lived experiences of personal current stories from a much broader, alive, diverse point of view. It also required that I, the faculty member, not be threatened by disagreements and critique, rather excited, open, and willing to learn from them. Actually, my personal/professional experience was and is "appreciative" and "grateful" for the students and their differing views. This process informed everyone and allowed new learning in a more contemporary framework of current social discourse of the time.

This personal teaching moment reflection captures some of the ingredients I honor and recommend to educators, both new and experienced—they include:

- Taking time.
- Listening.
- Creating open space—where students are encouraged to challenge, to disagree, to ask questions that may seem basic; I tell students "if you

do not challenge the education and thinking, then your education is not worth anything." Students need to be encouraged to translate the theory, the facts, the knowledge, the information into personal meaning and understanding that become purposive and whole for them.

▓ Creating safe trusting space—within the environmental field, the room, the emotional context along with the content—the wise educator does so in ways that engage the student actively, creatively, passionately in personal ways, so the distant knowledge and technical, factual information become personal knowledge; they own the understanding in ways that are whole for them.

This insight and wisdom for an educator is to understand self and your own talents and gifts and foibles; use authentic self in the teaching moments; do not try to be someone you are not.

The most effective teacher is the authentic teacher/person. We teach who we are, not just what we know.

It is a wise educator who knows that:

▓ Information is not knowledge;
▓ Knowledge is not understanding;
▓ Understanding is not necessarily wisdom, (that is, knowledge that is integrated into personal grasping /meaning, and becomes personal knowledge.

In summary, my advice/reflection for nursing education and nurse educators is to be awake to students and open to new learning from them, new emancipatory pedagogies and practices which evolve and emerge from co-creative process, drawing upon the combined talents and gifts of the whole. It is a wise educator who:

Creates a community of caring within the classroom and clinical setting; Invites authentic dialogue and questioning/processing of all the content into personal/professional experiences; "Sees" and respects the inner life experiences of the students and patients alike; Honors the inner subjective work of learning, beyond content per se, but integrated knowing/being/doing/becoming as one act; Helps students to model their best self and highest ethical ideals for themselves, even if they cannot see it for themselves at the moment; Practice caring and love in your life and learning beyond the classroom.

A small teaching example: I start all my classes (and my speaking presentations) by a heart-centering breathing exercise; cultivating a pause, in the moment to shift the field, becoming mindful of "being present in this moment"; to themselves and listening within to what they are there to learn, to give and receive in this moment of time, to appreciate themselves and the privilege of learning together.

This simple, brief centering exercise creates safe space and invites them into a personal reflective practice mode to be authentically present, it connects everyone in a common field; it is a method that can be repeated again and again in any situation. In turn you are modeling an emancipatory pedagogy and a clinically relevant practice of learning how to be "present," beyond just physical presence.

These are small but purposive tips as a career educator in human caring and nursing. If any nurse educator takes these reflections into their life learnings and teachings, I am convinced nursing education and human caring in education and practice will be strengthened and sustained for self, as well as the succeeding generations of nursing students.

REFERENCES

American Association of Colleges of Nurses. (2008). *The Essentials of Baccalaureate Education for Professional Nursing Practice. Retrieved from wwww.aacn. nche.edu/education-resources/baccessentials08.pdf*

American Association of Colleges of Nursing. (2012). Retrieved from www.aacn. nche.edu/

Alcantara, E. (2009). Nursing theorist: Martha Rogers. Retrieved from http://www. scribd.com

Benner, P. (1984). *From novice to expert: Excellence and power in clinical nursing practice*. Menlo Park, CA: Addison-Wesley.

Blaise, K., Hayes, J., Kozier, B., & Erb, G. (2006). *Theoretical foundation of professional nursing practice*. Upper Saddle River, NJ: Prentice-Hall, Inc.

Carper, B. (1978). Fundamental patterns of knowing in nursing. *Advances in Nursing Science, 1*, 33–54.

Coll, J. E., & Draves, P. (2009). Traditional age students: Worldviews and satisfaction with advising: A homogeneous study of student and advisors. *College Student Affairs Journal, 27*(2), 215–223.

Dickoff, J., James, P., & Wiedenbach E. (1968a). Theory in a practice discipline, part I. *Nursing Research, 17*:415–435.

Dickoff, J., & James, P. (1968). A Theory of Theories: A Position Paper, *Nursing Research, 17*: 197–203.

Johns, C. (1995). Framing learning through reflection within Carper's fundamental ways of knowing in nursing. *Journal of Advanced Nursing, 22*(2): 226–234. doi:10.1046/j.1365-2648.1995.22020226.x

Henderson, V. (1966). *The nature of nursing: A definition and its implications for practice, research, and education*. Riverside, NJ: Macmillan.

Kolcaba, K. (2001). Evolution of the mid range theory of comfort for outcomes research. *Nursing Outlook, 49*(2), 86–92.

Kolcaba, K. Y. (1994). A theory of holistic comfort for nursing. *Journal of Advanced Nursing, 19*(6), 1178–1184.

Leininger, M., & McFarland, M. (2002). *Transcultural nursing: Concepts, theories, research and practice* (3rd ed.). San Francisco, CA: McGraw-Hill.

Mishell, M. H., (1990). Reconceptualization of the uncertainty in illness theory. *Journal of Nursing Scholarship*, Winter; *22*(4):256–262.

Mishel, M. H. (1988). Uncertainty in illness. Image: *Journal of Nursing Scholarship, 20*:225–231.

Neuman, B. (1982). The Neuman health-care systems model: A total approach to client care. In B. Neuman (Ed.), *The Neuman systems model: Application to nursing education and practice* (pp. 8–29). Norwalk, CT: Appleton-Century-Crofts.

Newman, M. (2010). Health as expanding consciousness. Retrieved on November 13, 2010, from health as expanding consciousness: http://www.healthasexpanding consciousness.org/home/

Neuman's Theory. (2012). Retrieved from www.neumann.edu/academics/under-grad/nursing/model.asp

National Council of State Board of Nursing (NCSBN). (2012). https://www.ncsbn.org/

National League for Nursing. (2012). Retrieved from www.nln.org/

Nursing Theories. (2011). A companion to nursing theories and models. Retrieved from http://currentnursing.com/nursing_theory/Henderson.html

Orlando, I. J. (1961). The dynamic nurse-patient relationship: Function, process and principles. New York: G. P. Putman's Sons. [Reprinted 1990, New York: National League for Nursing.]

Orem, D. E. (1971). Nursing: Concept of practice. New York: McGraw-Hill.

Peplau, H. E. (1952). *Interpersonal relations in nursing*. New York: Putnam.

Rogers, M. E. (1989). *An introduction to the theoretical basis of nursing*. Philadelphia, PA: F.A. Davis.

Rogers, (1970). An Introduction to the Theoretical Bases of Nursing. Philadelphia: FA Davis

Ruland, C. M., & Moore, S. M., (1998). Theory construction based on standards of care: A proposed theory of the peaceful end of life. *Nursing Outlook, 44*(4), 169–175.

Taylor, S., & Renpenning, K. (2011). *Self-care science, nursing theory & evidence-based practice*. New York: Springer Publishing Company.

Walker, L., & Avant, K (2005). *Strategies for theory construction* (4th ed.). Upper Saddle River, NJ: Pearson/Prentice Hall.

Watson, J. (1979). Nursing: The Philosophy and Science of Caring. Boston: Little, Brown, and Co.

Watson, J. (2005). *Caring science as sacred science.* Philadelphia, PA: FA Davis.

Watson, J. (2009). Caring science and human caring theory: Transforming personal and professional practices of nursing and health care. *Journal of Health and Human Services Administration, 31*(4), 466–482.

PART III

Role of Faculty in a College/University

CHAPTER 13

Rank, Tenure, and Promotion

"Don't aim for success if you want it; just do what you love and believe in, and it will come naturally."

— DAVID FROST

OBJECTIVES

After reading this chapter, the reader will be able to
- Describe the four main faculty ranks
- Understand the importance of tenure
- Understand how to achieve tenure
- Discuss issues of tenure
- Describe the process of evaluation
- Discuss the process for promotion

INTRODUCTION

This chapter will focus on rank, tenure, and promotion. In the world of academe there is a specific set of criteria that faculty must meet in order to be eligible for each rank. Depending on one's past experience and level of education, an educator is assigned a specific rank when hired. To be eligible to advance to higher rank, faculty must have taught for the specified number of years and demonstrate through excellence in teaching, service, and scholarship that criteria for advancement to the next level have been met. This system and the process are quite formal. For an individual to be considered for promotion to the next faculty rank or for tenure, faculty must meet criteria and follow specific application guidelines as detailed in the faculty handbook of their academic institution. More rigorous criteria must be met to be eligible for tenure and when being promoted from the rank of associate to full professor. Full professor has more requirements than the other ranks.

FACULTY RANKS

The four main ranks in academia include:

1. The entry level of instructor
2. The second level of assistant professor
3. The third level of associate professor
4. The final level of full professor

To progress from one level to the next, faculty must demonstrate a certain level of proficiency in teaching, service, and scholarship, and demonstrate continued development as an educator and a scholar. Most new full-time educators begin at the instructor level. The title may vary, depending on the institution: lecturer, clinical instructor, or tenure track instructor. Each academic setting has individual requirements and may utilize the American Association of University Professors (AAUP) guidelines when creating polices on rank, tenure, and promotion. In an associate degree program faculty may be hired with a bachelor's degree with the understanding that a master's degree in nursing will be earned within a set timeframe. The following explanation of ranks pertains to baccalaureate nursing programs:

- Instructor level requires master's degree if hired for a tenure track position, expectations are that a doctoral degree will be earned within a specified timeframe. At the instructor level the major emphasis is on teaching and developing oneself as an expert teacher. The instructor will be required to participate in some type of service and scholarly activity but most of his/her time will be spent on teaching.
- The full-time lecturer or clinical instructor does not qualify for tenure but may be promoted to a higher rank based on teaching, service, and scholarship. They have a specific assignment and spend most of their time teaching.
- The assistant professor rank requires previous teaching experience, a master's degree, and enrollment in a doctoral program. Faculty at this rank spends most of his/her time in formal teaching activities but is expected to participate in scholarly activities, and become more involved in service activities.
- The associate professor rank requires a doctoral degree in addition to a specified amount of teaching experience, significant scholarship, and evidence of substantial service. The associate professor is expected to continue developing teaching skills; to participate in substantial scholarly activities such as grant funded research, publish widely, and have a substantial record of service to the college and community.
- A full professor must be an expert teacher, have at least 12 years of teaching experience at the college level, have contributed substantially in a scholarly way, and have an extensive record of service to both the college and the community. Most colleges and universities do not hire new faculty into the rank of full professor so they join at the associate degree level and after a specified period of time may apply for promotion to full professor.

In general, with each advancing rank there is an increase in salary. Furthermore, the expectations of teaching, service, and scholarship become more demanding. It is important to develop and maintain a portfolio of significant accomplishments and achievements. Each new faculty member will want to review the faculty handbook very carefully to become well-informed about the expectations the role. Each academic setting is unique and will have different expectations for faculty roles and responsibilities. For example, in the university setting you will be required to conduct research and may also be expected to obtain external funding for your research. At the college setting more emphasis is placed on the teaching role: while research is required at the associate and full professor ranks, it may not be necessary to obtain external funding. These are all important issues to understand when applying for a first teaching job. When seeking positions, be sure to read the expectations carefully and make sure all the requirements can be met. For example, do not apply for a position of associate professor when clearly you cannot meet the requirements of this role. It is important to note that some colleges/universities will count some adjunct teaching credits towards a candidate's years of teaching. In some schools, for example, 18 credits of adjunct teaching will be equivalent to one year of teaching. Sufficient adjunct credits may elevate the candidate's eligibility for the rank of assistant professor instead of instructor. Become fully informed about the requirements for eligibility for each faculty rank and analyze your own achievements and standing within those ranks. Upon hire, a one-year contract is offered that states rank, salary, and teaching load of the position. Contracts usually are offered for one or two years until tenure is achieved. The contract year may begin in September and end in August (twelve months) or may be a nine-month contract. If a full-year contract, a new contract will be offered every January. Always read the contract carefully before signing and returning it.

THE NURSE EDUCATOR'S WORK WEEK

The typical week of a nurse educator requires approximately 35–40 hours/week and to be at the college 4 days per week. There is usually one day off during the week for course preparation. Most undergraduate faculty teach 12 credits per semester; this is known as faculty load. Typical college courses are 3 or 4 credits but some may be less or more. In theory courses each credit equals 50–60 minutes of instruction. Clinical courses may be 1 credit for every 2 hours of instruction. Your workload may be as follows:

Med-Surg theory course: 4 credits (Tuesdays and Thursdays 9–11)
Med-Surg clinical course: 4 credits (Wednesdays 7–3)
Health Assessment course: 2 credits (Thursdays 12–2)
Pharmacology course: 2 credits (Thursdays 9–11)
Faculty Meetings: Every Monday 9–12

Prep time (prep, grading assignments, developing exams, etc.)
2 hours for every hour of instruction: 12 × 2 = 24 hours/week
Office hours: 4 hours per week/Tuesdays and Thursdays 12–2
Total hours per week: 47 hours (may vary based on amount of prep time)

This is a sample and may vary based on the academic setting. Preparation time will vary based on past experience with subject matter. The first time you teach a course requires the most prep time. Faculty may decide to grade assignments and exams at home or in their office. So the total hours per week will be divided between home and office. You will also need time to participate in scholarship and service. The faculty role is very demanding but it does offer a degree of flexibility in regards to prep time and other activities.

TENURE

Tenure is referred to as "permanence of appointment" and is granted to faculty after they have been teaching for at least seven years and have demonstrated excellence in teaching, scholarship, and service. Tenure also protects faculty members and enables them to function more independently in their research and thinking. Prior to initiation of tenure, many faculty were subject to lack of freedom of speech and thinking and were limited in their selection of research. Administrators might tell faculty to change grades or pass a failing student, especially if their family was influential or major financial contributors to the college or university. If faculty did not comply they would be fired. Tenure helps to protect faculty by ensuring academic freedom to faculty who have earned tenure or are on a tenure-track line. The following statement is from the AAUP website: *Academic Tenure*

After the expiration of a probationary period, teachers or investigators should have permanent or continuous tenure, and their service should be terminated only for adequate cause, except in the case of retirement for age, or under extraordinary circumstances because of financial exigencies.

In the interpretation of this principle it is understood that the following represents acceptable academic practice:

1. The precise terms and conditions of every appointment should be stated in writing and be in the possession of both institution and teacher before the appointment is consummated.
2. Beginning with appointment to the rank of full-time instructor or a higher rank, the probationary period should not exceed seven years, including within this period full-time service in all institutions of higher education; but subject to the proviso that when, after a term of probationary service of more than three years in one or more institutions, a teacher is called to another institution, it may be agreed in writing that the new appointment is for a probationary period of not more than four years, even though thereby the person's total probationary period in the academic profession

is extended beyond the normal maximum of seven years. Notice should be given at least one year prior to the expiration of the probationary period if the teacher is not to be continued in service after the expiration of that period.

3. During the probationary period a teacher should have the academic freedom that all other members of the faculty have.

4. Termination for cause of a continuous appointment, or the dismissal for cause of a teacher previous to the expiration of a term appointment, should, if possible, be considered by both a faculty committee and the governing board of the institution. In all cases where the facts are in dispute, the accused teacher should be informed before the hearing in writing of the charges and should have the opportunity to be heard in his or her own defense by all bodies that pass judgment upon the case. The teacher should be permitted to be accompanied by an advisor of his or her own choosing who may act as counsel. There should be a full stenographic record of the hearing available to the parties concerned. In the hearing of charges of incompetence the testimony should include that of teachers and other scholars, either from the teacher's own or from other institutions. Teachers on continuous appointment who are dismissed for reasons not involving moral turpitude should receive their salaries for at least a year from the date of notification of dismissal whether or not they are continued in their duties at the institution.

5. Termination of a continuous appointment because of financial exigency should be demonstrably bona fide (AAUP, 2006, p. 4).

The American Association of University Professors is an organization that helps to define and ensure professional standards and values of higher education, such as academic freedom and tenure (AAUP, 2012). It is a wonderful resource for new and seasoned faculty. The subject of tenure has recently received a lot of attention and there are proponents and opponents of the significance of tenure in the life of an academician. Balogun, Sloan, and Germain (2006) conducted a study on the proportion of nurse educators and allied health educators who were tenured and found that in allied health, the tenure rates were 47% and for nurse educators it was 35%. Some of the reasons cited for the low level of tenure are the heavy teaching/clinical workload of allied health and nurse educators. Furthermore, many of these faculty do not understand tenure, especially nurse educators who are from other countries. Another issue addressed by Mignor (2000) is the fact that nursing is somewhat of a newcomer to academe and nurse educators begin their careers in a clinical setting and are not acculturated to the nuance of a faculty role in an academic setting. Balogun et al. (2006) surveyed deans from nursing and allied health and 77% of them identified teaching as main criteria for tenure, while 25% of them identified scholarship, and fewer than 5% identified service. However, they also found that, currently, scholarship is the main factor in tenure decisions in research-based universities and is becoming more important in tenure decisions. Another issue with tenure relates to changes in the economy. Shaw and Maidment (2010) discuss the current state of the economy in relation to decreased tenure track positions. Since the 1970s, the percent of tenured faculty has dropped from 57% to 35%. Furthermore, many leaders in industry and business do not have a good understanding of tenure and some feel it protects teachers who are incompetent and teaching outdated material (p. 2). Although there is controversy surrounding tenure many faculty are eager to obtain tenure track positions in hopes of achieving tenure at their academic organizations.

The three main areas that are evaluated in tenure decisions are teaching, scholarship, and service. In many academic settings, teaching is the main expectation of educators (Billings & Halsted, 2009). To achieve tenure, faculty must demonstrate progressive improvement in teaching skills with the expectation that the candidate will become an "expert teacher" in their field. Many factors influence the tenure decision and include:

- Achievement of student outcomes based on exams, grades, and pass rates in addition to student evaluations are extremely important indicators.
- Peer evaluations and administrative reviews are also considered; every year faculty are reviewed by several peers.
- In many schools student evaluations play a significant role in the tenure decision.
- Scholarship is considered in tenure decisions. Scholarship may be in the form of research that is conducted individually or with a group. Research that receives external funding and is published in a peer-reviewed journal is expected in a research-based setting (AAUP, 1999). Publications of books, chapters, or articles are also required. It is important to get published in peer-reviewed or refereed journals, although it is acceptable to publish in other venues, too. Presenting at a conference, completing book reviews, or serving as a peer reviewer for a journal is another good way to develop a track record of scholarly activity.
- Service is the activity faculty participates in without monetary compensation. This includes serving on committees at the academic setting and being involved in community organizations. Although service may not be the priority area, it is still important to participate in some type of service as it is still viewed favorably. However, as a new faculty member it is best to focus as much as possible on your role development as a teacher. (Refer to Chapters 1, 16, and 17 for additional information.)

Although there are no specific guidelines for balancing teaching, scholarship, and service, faculty typically may plan to organize time devoted to these three roles with the highest percentage of time devoted to teaching. For example, one time management plan is to spend 80% of time teaching, 10% of time on scholarship, and 10% of time participating in service activities. It is wise to follow guidelines that are set forth by your academic setting. There are examples when faculty may be required to serve on a school of nursing committee and a college-wide committee. These types of committees help to meet service expectations and also serve as useful way to learn about the new organization and to meet faculty and staff. As a first-year teacher, scholarship likely will be related to becoming fully informed about the teaching role and researching the literature to learn more about the content to be taught. Enrollment in a doctoral program is usually considered a fulfillment of scholarly activity expectations. The important point is to demonstrate continued growth and development.

Most tenure-track positions offer two options: a 3- to 4-year line or a 7-year line. Faculty who have experience and have already earned their doctoral degree will usually sign a three/four-year contract. This gives them time to become acclimated to their new setting and to build their dossier. If you are a new faculty with limited academic teaching experience and are enrolled or planning to enroll in a doctoral program, you will probably sign a 7-year contract. Although this may seem like a lot of time, it goes by very quickly. Time is needed to develop as an educator and to earn the doctoral degree. Once hired into this type of role, develop a plan with long- and short-range goals in the areas of teaching, scholarship, and service. Also be sure to maintain a clear and concise record of all of your achievements and accomplishments. Do this every semester so when the time comes to submit a tenure application, the required information and documentation needed to demonstrate growth in teaching, scholarship, and service will be organized and complete. Tenure is not automatic! Each faculty must follow the specific guidelines of the organization when preparing the tenure application. Once completed, the application usually is submitted to the Rank, Tenure, and Salary Committee for review.

TENURE PORTFOLIO OR DOSIER

Most likely you will be required to develop a portfolio or dossier to demonstrate that you have met the criteria for tenure. The portfolio includes a curriculum vitae (CV) and three separate executive summaries of accomplishments and achievements in teaching, scholarship, and service. Supporting evidence must be included for each of the three areas in a portfolio or dossier (Billings, 2008). Think carefully about achievements so nothing is overlooked. For example, include work devoted to developing a new course or part of a new course; include teaching an innovative or new online course, or development of a new way to teach using technology; include being awarded a grant, or publishing articles; include presentations at conferences; serving on all committees with specifics about your role, participation, and accomplishments; include invitations to speak at a conference, or review a manuscript; and lastly, include samples of your work. You may be required to include your student and peer evaluations or they may be submitted by administration. It takes time to develop a professional and well written portfolio. Take the time necessary to substantiate how you have met all requirements. Most often, if all the requirements for teaching, scholarship, and service are met and there are no financial hardships at your college/university, you should receive tenure. Some tips to help ensure your success include taking the following steps:

- Be sure to start your application process early so you have plenty of time to obtain all the required documents.
- Request a letter of support from your dean, department chair, or both.
- Have your mentor or a senior faculty member review and critique your portfolio.
- Carefully follow the guidelines and meet the deadline for submission.
- Find out what options you have if you are unable to complete your doctoral program in time. Some colleges/universities may grant a 1-year extension or may offer another solution.
- Be proactive! If you do not receive tenure, you will not be able to keep your position and will have to leave when your current contract expires.
- If you do not receive tenure you may appeal the decision. If you choose to appeal be sure to read the guidelines on how to submit a formal appeal.

Some faculty also receive promotion to the next rank at the same time but this depends on the specific policy of your organization.

Once tenure if received, you will have a certain level of security but you will still be expected to continue to develop as a teacher and scholar and to participate in service activities. You will also be subject to periodic post-tenure review. Once you receive tenure it cannot be taken away. However, in extreme circumstances you may still be let go from your position.

PROMOTION

Promotion in the academic setting is a formal process that is similar to the tenure process. With each advance in rank, the faculty role becomes more prestigious and there is a significant salary increase. In some academic settings higher ranking faculty participate more in research and various administrative roles. Similar to tenure, promotion is not automatic and faculty must formally apply for promotion. To be considered for promotion you must have a record of teaching effectiveness, required teaching experience, academic experience, professional experience, professional activities, scholarship, and service. In addition a record of positive peer, student, and administrative evaluations is extremely important. Evaluations are done on a continual basis throughout the year. Administrative and peer evaluations are usually completed in the fall semester prior to contract renewals. Most often you will have an opportunity to select your peer evaluators. You may be required to have one peer evaluate your teaching, another peer evaluate your scholarship, and a third peer to evaluate your service. Peer evaluations are done by senior faculty who are tenured. When these evaluations are completed you will meet with the reviewer and receive a copy of their evaluation. This evaluation is done in a spirit of collegiality in an effort to help you to continue to improve.

Student evaluations are usually completed for all courses. Although you do not see the student evaluations you will be given feedback in aggregate form. You should use these evaluations to see what students think you are doing well and what areas they think you need to improve.

When completing the application for promotion specific guidelines should be followed with all the completed paperwork. This also entails developing a binder or portfolio of your accomplishments and achievements in the areas of teaching, scholarship, and service. In order to be considered for promotion you must meet all the requirements of the particular rank. For example, an associate professor must have a doctoral degree and a record of scholarship, and a certain number of years of experience. Some institutions require an interval of a certain number of years between promotions to give the candidate ample time to participate in additional teaching, scholarship, and service opportunities. It is important to demonstrate continued growth, excellence, and achievements as you progress from one rank to the next. So if you have not had the opportunity to develop a record of scholarship you should wait to apply for promotion. You will also need a letter of support from your department head or chairperson. You should always have your mentor or senior faculty member review your application and portfolio as you want to make a good impression. When being considered for promotion you usually do not get to meet in person with the committee so your portfolio needs to demonstrate that you meet all the expected requirements for the next rank. If you are not approved for promotion you will stay in your current rank until you feel you are ready to apply again for promotion.

SUMMARY

This chapter focused on faculty rank tenure, and promotion. The importance of teaching, scholarship, and service in relation to tenure and promotion was discussed. The development of the portfolio and examples of what to include in one were also discussed. Being aware of the specific guidelines and seeking input from mentors and senior faculty is very important and new faculty should develop a short- and long-term plan in regards to tenure and promotion.

DISCUSSION QUESTIONS

1. Discuss the four types of faculty rank and how they are different.
2. Discuss the significance of tenure.
3. Identify some current issues with tenure.
4. Describe the process for tenure.
5. Identify specific areas in teaching, learning, and scholarship that will help you achieve tenure and promotion.

SUGGESTED LEARNING ACTIVITIES

▪ Develop a plan with short- and long-term goals based on a seven-year tenure contract.
▪ Make a chart for teaching, scholarship, and service that lists all of your accomplishments to date.
▪ Review the literature on tenure and develop a position paper that is for or against tenure. You must support your position with the literature and current research.

REFERENCES

American Association of University Professors (2012) retrieved from www.aaup.org/
American Association of University Professors. (2006). 1940 *Statement of principles on academic freedom and tenure with 1970 interpretive comments.* Retrieved from http://www.aaup.org › *AAUP* › *Issues in Higher Ed* › *Academic Freedom*
American Association of Colleges of Nursing. (1999). *Position statement on defining scholarship for the discipline of nursing.* Retrieved from http://www.AACN.com
Balogun, J. A., Sloan, P. E., & Germain, M. (2006). Determinants of tenure in allied health and nursing education. *Journal of Advanced Nursing, 56*(5), 532–541. doi: 10.1111/j.1365–2648.2006.04045.x.
Billings, D. (2008). Developing your career as a nurse educator. The professional Portfolio. *Journal of Continuing Education in Nursing, 39*(12), 532–533.
Billings, D. M., & Halstead, J. A. (2009). *Teaching in nursing: A guide for faculty* (3rd ed.). Philadelphia, PA: W. B. Saunders.
Mignor, D. (2000). Who is going to teach undergraduate clinicals? *Nursing Forum, 35*(3), 21.
Shaw, D., & Maidment, F. (2010). Getting tenure in a down economy. *Journal of College Teaching & Learning, 7*(12), 1–4.

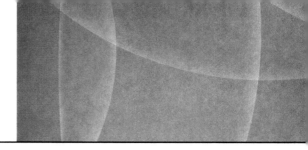

The Faculty Role in the College/
University Setting

RUTH A. WITTMANN-PRICE, PhD, RN, CNS, CNE

COMPLETING A TERMINAL DEGREE AND PRODUCING scholarly publications are the nemesis of many nurse educators. Nurse educators are clinical experts and very adept teachers, but clinical expertise and classroom proficiency are not the only criteria that are evaluated in the academic realm. This reflective piece is related to my own experience as a faculty member and department chair, and is written to assist others to better understand academic expectations and how to reflect on how they fit with personal career goals.

First, understand that by accepting an academic job, you have consented to "play by the rules" of the collegiate team. The rulebook is the faculty handbook, especially the section about promotion and tenure, and in order to play by the rules the nurse educator must know the rulebook inside and out. This is imperative in order to develop a realistic career trajectory.

The faculty handbook outlines the criteria for promotion and tenure in slightly ambiguous terms. It reads, "For promotion to associate professor candidates should have a terminal degree in the discipline" (FMU, 2010, p. 24). The word "should" leaves room for misunderstanding. Many times nurse educators interpret these purposeful gray areas as flexible criteria but unfortunately this can be a dangerous interpretation.

There are several reasons why criteria often are worded this ambiguously. One reason may historical: there may have been associate professors without terminal degrees who were valued and productive employees of the academic institution. Another reason may be that an amazing expert in a discipline may be hired and promoted to this rank, and even though they do not have a terminal degree, they possess other qualifications such as having published three best-selling books on the subject. The ambiguous wording usually does not mean that someone is *likely* to be promoted without a terminal degree. Any nurse educator who is applying for promotion or tenure should be certain they have reached and exceeded the criteria listed in every area of teaching, scholarship/research, and service before applying. Applying for promotion or tenure with any significant doubts about meeting promotion and tenure criteria can be a devastating career move.

The best method of avoiding pressure when the promotion and tenure clock is ticking prematurely is to be selective when job hunting or changing positions. Clearly understand the types of academic settings that are available and choose a setting that fits your current skill sets, promotes advancement, but does not push you into a promotion corner if you are not ready. Know if the institution where you are applying or if the department you are applying within is a research-intensive university, or if it's a college with a clinical track that does not require research to qualify for promotion. If teaching is your passion, search for an institution whose primary mission is teaching. In any position, know how much publication is expected and what types of manuscripts are expected, such as data-driven, peer-reviewed articles in high impact journals, or if chapters and/or books are acceptable (Wittmann-Price, 2012).

Often nurse educators are anxious to land their first academic position, but they may enter into the position not knowing sufficient background about the academic system and its particular expectations. Being unaware of the organizational structure, benefits, and promotion expectations increases the likelihood an unsuccessful transition. Remember, since there is a shortage of nurse educators, you can afford to be selective and find an academic position that is a good fit for you.

Before accepting employment, or when choosing to change positions, research and analyze all the institutional information carefully. Nurse educators should ***consider expectations realistically***. For example, if a position places you on a six-year tenure track and you have not started back for your doctorate when you accept the position, you should understand that the average PhD takes five to seven years to complete.

Academia is a wonderful place to work, but a much different culture than hospitals. Even though nurses' work is renowned in the clinical sector, most practice is not evaluated per se in academia. Nor do most academic administrators consider the fact, that while other academic professors were gaining expertise in teaching, scholarship/research, and service, nurse educators were practicing full-time and acquiring advanced degrees part-time.

Although much of this sounds harsh, I am writing it because I have been, and have witnessed nurse educators who have been, dehumanized within an academic system. The goal of this reflective paper is to share my insights to protect future nurse educators from being devalued. Each one of us is an incredibly hard worker who is passionate about educating the much-needed next generation of nurses. Be sure that you understand your career goals, and then match them realistically with an academic position that will best support you in fulfilling those goals, as this "match" is crucial to your academic success!

REFERENCES

Francis Marion University (FMU). (2010). *Faculty handbook.*

Wittmann-Price, R. A. (2012). *Fast facts for developing a nursing academic portfolio.* New York, NY: Springer Publishing.

CHAPTER 14

Collegiality, Service, and Leadership Roles of the Educator

"Do not go where the path may lead, go instead where there is no path and leave a trail."

—RALPH WALDO EMERSON

OBJECTIVES

After reading this chapter, the reader will be able to
- Understand the significance of collegiality in academia
- Discuss specific areas of collegiality
- Understand the importance of service in the life of a faculty member
- Describe ways to meet the expectation of service in academe
- Discuss possible leadership roles for nurse educators

COLLEGIALITY AND ACADEMIA

The word "collegiality" often brings to mind the following connotations: colleague, respect, interpersonal relationships, teamwork, and positive working relationships. All of these words and phrases share the common meaning of being able to work well with colleagues in the workplace setting. Some examples of collegiality are collaboration, mentoring and precepting of new faculty, professionalism, and treating colleagues with respect. Balsmeyer, Haubrich, and Quinn (1996) posit:

> The behaviors synonymous with collegiality are often unwritten and, therefore, remain ambiguous and obscure to many nurse educators. However, judgments about a faculty member's relationships with colleagues may be an important consideration in annual performance reviews or decisions regarding promotion or the granting of tenure. (p. 264)

Behaviors that are not collegial include being argumentative, bullying, gossiping, shame and blame, and belittling others. Collegiality is especially significant in academic settings with a small number of faculty. These faculty must work closely together to develop curriculum and policies and may even be required to team teach. When faculty do not have good interpersonal relationships job satisfaction and productivity may decrease. Collegiality is valued in academia and many feel it should be included in the formal evaluation process. Currently it is included in tenure and promotion decisions but falls under the umbrella of teaching, scholarship, and service. Many academicians are hesitant to include it formally in decisions of tenure and promotion because it is somewhat elusive and difficult to measure. Furthermore, many academics worry that adding this to the triad of teaching, scholarship, and service may impinge on academic freedom. Furthermore, some feel it may prevent tenure and promotion as it is subjective and may be judged based on personal feelings towards one another. For example, Haag (2005) discussed the issue of collegiality and discrimination against minority populations. In the past it has been very difficult for faculty to win an appeal when the decision not to promote or grant tenure was based on issues relating to collegiality. Currently, the professoriate and the AAUP recognize the significance of collegiality in academia but are hesitant to recommend including collegiality in the formal evaluation process (Johnston, Schimmel, & O'Hara, 2010). Although it may not be a separate entity in the evaluation process it is still considered in decisions of tenure and promotion. As a new faculty member you will want to try to establish good working relationships with your peers. Most faculty will be very welcoming and help you to acclimate to your new role. However, there may be one or two faculty who are not very supportive. The important thing is to try to develop positive relationships and learn as much as you can from the more experienced faculty who are interested in helping you. Hopefully, you will not experience bullying in your workplace. However, if it does happen be sure to take a proactive approach and discuss it with your mentor, dean, or department head. There is usually a zero-tolerance policy for bullying so do not be intimidated. Johnston et al. (2010) support the inclusion of collegiality in the formal process of evaluation and based on the results of their study posit that utilizing a model of collegiality may address many of the concerns of evaluating collegiality. Furthermore, during their review of the literature they found that most faculty view collegiality more favorably than workload and it also has a significant impact on job satisfaction. However, because of ambiguity a formal evaluation tool is recommended to give clear guidelines and expectations. Russell (2010) found that collegiality in senior faculty was highly correlated with job satisfaction and productivity. Since senior faculty comprise more than 50% of all faculty it is important to identify and address issues that increase retention. In an earlier study Pollicino (1996) found that collegiality between faculty and administration was significantly related to job satisfaction in faculty. In summary, collegiality is an important issue for faculty especially in relationship to job satisfaction and retention. However, because of ambiguity and subjectivity fair and objective methods must be developed to include this factor in formal evaluation. So what does this all mean to you as a new educator? It means that you need to consider the impact of collegiality in decisions of tenure and promotion. Developing positive working relationships should be one of your goals. Things to be cognizant of are behaviors in meetings where controversial topics may be discussed. It is important to stay in control and present your views in a professional manner. Unfortunately, gossiping may occur in any organization and it is important not to partake in this type of negative behavior. It is also important to collaborate and be a team player. Try to volunteer for things such as open houses or task forces. You want to try to establish good citizenship with all faculty, staff, and administrators in your department and the entire college community. There are many events that take place during the year and although they may not be mandatory you should try to attend at least a few throughout the year. You also want to establish good relationships in the community and with your clinical partners. Whether it is included formally or informally collegiality will have an impact on your tenure and promotion.

SERVICE

Service is a requirement of all faculty and there are many ways you can fulfill this requirement. Service is something that is considered "good for society" and includes your individual school or program, the college at large, the profession, and the community. It is also something that does not involve financial compensation. As a new faculty member you may meet the service criteria internally by joining committees or partaking in open houses. Jenkins (2006) posits that service is even more important in community colleges because there is less emphasis on scholarly work. Filetti (2009) states, "As an undergraduate state university that focuses on a liberal arts education, my university stresses excellence in teaching, scholarship and service, with the annual review of faculty counting teaching 50% scholarship 25% and service 25%" (p. 343). Although service is usually not weighed as heavily as teaching and scholarship it is still important and usually the expectation increases as you move up in rank. Furthermore, each organization is different so you need to understand what the expectations in your particular setting are for amount and types of service.

Types of service include:

- Committee membership (internal and external)
- Volunteering
- Mentoring
- Being a peer reviewer
- Advising student groups
- Serving as an editor
- Being part of an editorial board
- Becoming a board member
- Presenting at various locations

▪ Recruitment efforts for the program
▪ Serving on a task force or community board
▪ Service learning

The above items are just some of the areas where one might engage in service. It is important to note that some of these require an official appointment. Furthermore, in many programs committee membership is mandatory but is still viewed as service. For example, the nursing program may have several committees. These might include curriculum, program evaluation, and institutional resources. Depending on the policy of your academic setting you might be appointed to a committee, be allowed to self select, or be voted onto a committee. Membership in committees might be done on a rotating basis to give all faculty an opportunity to serve on a particular committee. Participating in these types of committees helps you to learn more about your program and your school. You also become better acquainted with your peers and develop collegial relationships. Chairing a committee is also a great experience although some feel because of potential controversial issues you should not be a committee chair until you are tenured.

Jenkins (2006) offers some advice for participating on committees:

▪ Make a point to attend every meeting, and if you have to miss one, be sure to send the head of the committee an email explaining why.
▪ Be an active, participating member but not the most vocal person at the table. When asked for your opinion, be honest yet tactful. Behave collegially toward everyone and avoid taking sides too soon—unless you really feel strongly about an issue and are sure you have chosen the right side.
▪ Volunteer, when appropriate, to lead a subcommittee or take on other tasks on behalf of the group. That way, your committee work can provide more than just short-term annual-report fodder. It can genuinely boost your career by helping you become a respected and influential member of the faculty (para. 9).

College-wide committees are another way to meet the expectation of service and also give you an opportunity to learn more about the college and meet faculty from different programs and departments. Some of the common college-wide programs include the Senate, Council of Faculty, Tenure Committee, and the Institutional Review Board. As a new faculty member you would not be eligible to sit on the Tenure Committee or the Institutional Review Board. There are also committees or task forces on various aspects of the college that you may be able to join. Depending on how your school is set up you may feel disconnected from the rest of the college or university and becoming involved can make a difference. It is important to form collegial relationships with faculty from different departments. This is especially the case in undergraduate nursing programs where your students will be taking some courses in liberal arts and sciences and you may be required to collaborate on joint projects or participate in team teaching.

Evaluating one's service is somewhat ambiguous as some types of service may be difficult to quantify. Filetti (2009) found that the value of service varies among academic settings. For example, in universities that require substantial research service may not even be considered. Another issue is how to measure and evaluate service. How does one decide which activity is given more weight? Neumann and Terosky (2007) posit "Service then has emerged, paradoxically, as necessary for the institutional welfare *and* as unacknowledged in faculty work lives. Unrecognized as a form of "real" faculty work, it is also underresearched as a "real" strand of the faculty career" (p. 284). Furthermore, they describe the process for evaluating service as something nebulous and point out that there are limited studies on this subject. Neumann and Terosky also found that faculty participated in more service after tenure and that the faculty felt it helped them to develop and to become more involved in the life of the institution. Hassna and Raza (2011) investigated the relationship of the triad of teaching, scholarship, and service and found a significant relationship between faculty teaching and service. Participating in service activities actually helped faculty to improve their teaching skills. A guideline with specific criteria and weight of particular areas should be developed so that faculty service is fair and balanced. As a new faculty member you may want to consult with your mentor on how to best meet the requirement of service (ASHE-ERIC Higher Education Report, 2003).

SERVICE AT THE PROGRAM LEVEL

Committee Membership

A common way for all faculty to participate in internal service is through membership and participation in program committees. Assignments to committees may be done in different ways and they all offer an opportunity for faculty, especially new faculty, to learn and contribute to the future direction of the program. Many schools also invite students to be non-voting observers of their committees. Members of committees spend time researching and reviewing current literature, research, and evidence so that they can be productive members of their committee. Sometimes, smaller task forces are created to address a particular issue. The mission, philosophy, and bylaws of the program or school along with licensing and accrediting standards guide the mission and format of a particular committee or task force. Attendance and minutes are always required and Robert's Rule of Order is often utilized to guide the meeting and maintain professional discourse. Committees usually meet at least once a month and are charged with a specific set of objectives. The committee structure is set up so that the committee does the work and votes on any changes as a group and then brings it to the entire faculty. Major changes are then approved by the dean, then the administration, and then if applicable the state. Minor changes are voted on by the faculty and it goes by majority rule but must follow the bylaws of your institution. There is usually a chairperson who is responsible for guiding the meeting and for bringing the decisions of the committee to the entire faculty and administration. Whenever a new change is presented it requires a vote by the full faculty and a quorum must be reached. Approval is based on majority rule and then most often requires administrative approval.

There are many ways to meet the expectation of service right in your own program. Because faculty in all types of programs play an important role in curriculum development, teaching and learning, and evaluation of program effectiveness committees are in place for faculty to do this important work. Most programs have several committees and faculty are divided among the committees. Because the curriculum belongs to the faculty there is usually a curriculum committee. This is an extremely important committee as the curriculum must be updated on a continual basis to reflect the integration of new concepts, technology, and standards. Members of this and other committees spend time researching and reviewing current literature, research, and evidence so that they can be productive members of the committee. Licensure and accreditation standards must also be considered when reviewing and revising the curriculum.

A committee on program effectiveness focuses on outcomes and develops evaluation methods on various parts of the program. These programs are guided by state and institutional guidelines, accrediting agencies, and ongoing evaluation (Gard, Flannigan, & Cluskey, 2004). Typical areas that are evaluated include specific programs, faculty, and clinical sites, in addition to overall program outcomes. Gard et al. (2004) state the program evaluation committee's role is to collect, analyze, store, and report on evaluation results. Based on their analysis and benchmarking data they develop plans for improvement.

Gard et al. (2004) state

Program evaluation serves several purposes:
- Maintaining quality
- Assessing curriculum and instruction
- Identifying areas of challenge
- Facilitating program improvement
- Providing data for reports to state agencies, accrediting agencies, and governing boards. (p. 179)

Collecting data on programs can be particularly challenging so one school developed a way to use technology and social media to increase participation in the evaluation process. Story et al. (2010) utilized emails, social media such as Facebook, and online evaluation tools such as Survey Monkey to collect important data from alumnus and found this was a very effective way to collect data. Serving on this type of committee can help new faculty become familiar with the accreditation process and the importance of collecting, analyzing, and utilizing data for program improvement.

Another committee may be the resource committee which is responsible for evaluating current resources and for making recommendations for improving, updating, or adding new resources. These resources relate to the resources faculty need to provide quality education and the resources students need to succeed in the program.

The search committee is another important committee. When positions become available the search committee screens potential applicants. They review the curriculum vitae or resumes and set up interviews. The committee is usually comprised of faculty and students and one faculty member is appointed as chair. Once the committee approves a candidate the recommendation is given to the dean or other appropriate person for the next step of the interview process. Faculty have a very significant role in selecting their future colleagues. Chairing a search committee is viewed as a prestigious role and most often requires a senior faculty member. As a new faculty member you may be asked to sit on a search committee.

College-wide committees include the tenure review committee, faculty council committee, and senate. These committees are charged with important areas of faculty life and represent the entire college. Faculty are usually voted onto these committees and serve for a specific term. Only tenured faculty are eligible to serve on the tenure committee. The role of the tenure committee is to review faculty contracts, and applications for tenure and promotion. This is an extremely important committee and is comprised of senior faculty members who represent different parts of the college. For example, there might be two representatives from nursing, two from arts and sciences, and two from the library. The committee reviews all the information and makes a recommendation to the administration on whether a faculty should be tenured, promoted, or have their contract renewed. This committee utilizes the evaluation of teaching, scholarship, and service in their decision-making process. As a new faculty member it is important to understand the role of this committee and to attend any informational sessions that are provided by these seasoned faculty members.

The faculty council is devoted to issues pertaining to faculty life. Any full-time faculty member can be voted on to this committee. Issues addressed by this committee include the faculty handbook and policies and procedures related to faculty such as workload, evaluation process, and faculty development. This is a good committee for new faculty to learn about the specific guidelines for faculty. As a rule you must be voted onto this committee by your faculty peers and will serve a specified term.

The senate is the governing body of the college and is usually comprised of faculty, staff, and administration. Representatives are voted by their peers to serve specific terms and work on improving all aspects of academic life. The purpose is to maintain shared governance and the senate creates policies and makes recommendations but final approval is usually granted by the president. The power and influence of the senate varies based on the philosophy of the academic institution. As a new faculty member becoming a senator is a great experience that will enable you to develop collegial relationships with many faculty and staff. You will also learn about the entire institution and will gain a better understanding of financial and governing bodies that influence academic institutions.

Service to the Community

There are many ways you can serve your community and the caveat is that it should relate to your area of expertise and not involve monetary rewards. You may choose to offer educational programs to various community agencies such as schools, churches, or senior citizen centers. You may be asked to serve as a consultant or expert on a particular topic. Serving on an editorial review board is a great experience. In this role you offer expert advice on content and future articles and direction of the journal or magazine. Becoming a peer reviewer, which can also be considered as a scholarly endeavor, is also highly recommended. Most of the journals seek voluntary peer reviewers and they give you specific guidelines for completing the review. You might serve on your community board or chair its health and human services committee. Visiting local middle schools and high schools to discuss the nursing profession and various health topics as part of community outreach is another option. Many schools become involved in community service projects for the underserved and you might join that effort or even serve as the faculty advisor. You might also consider writing a health column for your local newspaper. These are just a few of the possibilities. The important thing is to set realistic goals for yourself and to enjoy your work.

Service to the Profession

There are many professional organizations in nursing and it is important to hold membership in several of them. Many nursing faculty join organizations in their field of expertise. For example, a nurse educator who teaches transcultural nursing will join the Transcultural Nursing Society. Many schools have group membership in the American Association of Colleges of Nursing (AACN), the American Nurses Association (ANA), and the National League for Nurses (NLN). Thus when you join the faculty you automatically become a member of one of these organizations. The Honor Society of Nursing Sigma Theta Tau International is an organization that nurses are invited to join based on their academic achievements or contributions to the nursing profession. As a members of professional organizations you will have the opportunity to network and to collaborate with colleagues from around the world. You will also have an opportunity to become involved in committee work or task forces. You might also answer calls for abstracts for presentations at various conferences. These projects are subject to peer review and, because there is no financial compensation, may be considered both under the areas of scholarship and service. You may also be nominated to serve as an officer and represent your college or geographic area. As you become more experienced you might want to consider becoming an accreditor for CCNE or NLNAC (Rizzo Nikou, 2000, as cited in Scheetz, 2000). If you are interested in serving as an accreditor you can find more information on the respective websites regarding qualifications and application process. These positions are voluntary but are considered highly prestigious and are a wonderful learning opportunity. If you are selected you will attend a formal training program on how to serve as an accreditor. It truly is a wonderful learning experience and something all faculty should consider. All of these experiences will help you to meet the expectations of service and also contribute to your professional role development.

DEVELOPING A PLAN

There are so many wonderful opportunities for nurse educators to contribute to their programs, schools, community, and profession. Although requirements for service vary based on institution there are some guidelines for participating in service. For example, Rizzo Nikou (2000) states service hours should be 4–6 hours per month but that many faculty actually spend about 10 hours per month on service-related activities. Although many institutions do not specify specific type of service or amount of hours you should check with your dean or mentor, and review the faculty handbook. It is helpful to create a specific plan on how you will address the issue of service. Early on in your teaching career you will want to focus mostly on developing your role as a master teacher and will spend most of your time in this area. However, it is vital to be involved in at least one or two service-related activities. Just be careful not to take on too much responsibility. As you become more experienced, you will want to increase your service-related activities. There is a reciprocal relationship because many of these experiences will help you to develop your role as an educator and also demonstrate your collegiality. It is also a way to develop your portfolio and demonstrate your professionalism.

LEADERSHIP AND THE NURSE EDUCATOR ROLE

There are several areas where nurse educators may serve as leaders. This may include being a lead teacher, serving as the course coordinator, chairing a committee, or serving as a leader in a professional organization. Many nurse educators assume these types of leadership roles very early on in their academic career. Nurse educators have various backgrounds and many of them have previous leadership experience which helps to prepare them for these roles. The following quote by Eleanor Roosevelt, "A good leader inspires people to have confidence in the leader, a great leader inspires people to have confidence in themselves," captures the very essence of a leader. If you are invited to serve in a leadership capacity you will want to be knowledgeable about the various leadership theories (Bass, 1985) and consider your philosophy of leadership. A widely embraced style is transformational leadership. These leaders are often described as charismatic leaders who influence subordinates to meet the goals of an organization. They also help others realize their full potential, to understand the importance of their tasks, and to put the good of the organization above their personal need (Green, 2005). Kouzes and Posner (2007) have been studying leadership practices for over 25 years and have developed what they describe as the behaviors of an exemplary leader. The behaviors are: model the way, inspire a shared vision, challenge the process, enable others to act, and encourage the heart. There are many resources and role development seminars that can help you develop and refine your role as a leader.

Faculty members may also serve as the course coordinator for their theory/clinical courses. For example, a faculty member who teaches the theory portion of Foundations, or Med-Surg will often be the course coordinator for the theory and clinical components of the course. The responsibilities of the course coordinator are to develop the course syllabi, and outlines for both the theory and clinical courses. The course coordinator may also oversee the clinical adjuncts and may be responsible for orienting and evaluating their performance. Some course coordinators are also responsible for arranging their own clinical placements. This is a wonderful way to gain experience as a leader in the field of nursing education.

Committee work is a very important part of the academic role and you may be asked to chair a committee. This may be in a college-wide committee or a school of nursing committee. The specific role and responsibilities will vary based on the type of committee and your academic organization. Some of the responsibilities of the chair are to schedule meetings, develop the agendas, and lead the meetings. You may also be responsible for keeping records and reporting on the progress of your committee at larger meetings. This type of role requires leadership, organization, interpersonal skills, problem-solving, delegation, and an understanding of group dynamics. This type of responsibility may be very helpful in your tenure process and also demonstrates your commitment to the organization.

A future role for nurse educators may be to become a department chair, associate dean, or dean. These roles are often sought after by senior faculty and require extensive academic and leadership experience. If one of your goals is to become an administrator it is a good idea to develop a plan that will enable you to develop over time and to demonstrate your leadership abilities. There is often a progression of roles that begin with the role of department chair and then the assistant or associate role and eventually the role of dean. Teaching responsibilities vary among these types of positions. For example, most department chairs have a teaching assignment. However, the deans may not teach or may teach only one course per semester. If you are interested in this type of position, you will want to explore whether you will be able to return to your faculty role. Most academic settings will allow you to return to a faculty position. Volunteering for different leadership roles, such as chairing a committee or serving as a course coordinator, is a great way to gain experience for this type of role.

Leadership roles outside of academia involve administrative roles in accreditation agencies such as American Association of Colleges of Nurses or the National League for Nurses, or in one of the various professional organizations.

These roles require extensive experience and previous involvement with the organization. Often, potential candidates must be voted into one of these leadership roles. A good way to get involved is to be an active member and join task forces and committees so that you will learn more about the organization and get to network with the other members. These are highly visible roles and provide an opportunity for you to guide the profession in its current and future development.

Teaching a leadership course or integrating leadership theory is another role. Many nursing programs offer their students a leadership course or integrate leadership theory throughout the curriculum. If you are required to teach one of these courses you will want to become well versed in the various leadership theories.

In summary, many nurse educators will be called to serve as a leader in one capacity or another and there are many opportunities for serving as a leader. If you are interested in one of the many leadership roles it is important to have a sound knowledgebase on leadership and the related theories and to seek experiences where you can develop your leadership role.

SUMMARY

Collegiality and service are two important but somewhat ambiguous areas for all faculty. It is important to establish good working relationships and partake in various service related activities. All of these experiences will help you to learn and grow and develop your role as a respected academician. A future role as a leader in nurse education may also be something you aspire to achieve.

DISCUSSION QUESTIONS

1. Discuss the importance of collegiality in the life of an academician.
2. Compare and contrast behaviors related to positive and negative aspects of collegiality.
3. Discuss the importance of service in tenure and promotion.
4. Describe the four main areas that involve service.
5. List at least five different types of service and what they entail.

SUGGESTED LEARNING ACTIVITIES

- Make a list of all current service activities and your contributions.
- Interview a faculty member about their specific service activities and their views and advice on service to new faculty members.
- Select one area that you can participate in to count as service.
- Develop a plan with short- and long-term goals related to your service activities.

Leadership and Change: Risk and Accountability

GERALDINE (POLLY) BEDNASH, PhD, RN, FAAN

THE IDEA OF BEING A LEADER is filled with excitement, trepidation, and often some misperceptions about what being a leader entails. Heifetz and Linsky write in the *Harvard Business Review* that leadership is dangerous work in which you are like the point person in the infantry—out in front and often the one to take the first shot. However, leadership is an essential quality to advance health care in this nation, to advance our work as professionals, and to improve the quality of education, practice, and research in nursing.

Many individuals wonder if being a leader is an inherent trait that individuals are born with while others assert strongly that anyone can be taught to be a leader. I believe the answer is really somewhere in the middle. Any of us who have experienced the Myers-Briggs personality assessment know that humans come with a variety of potential to interact with others, to persuade, or to innovate. All of these are essential elements of leadership. So, clearly, if we all do not have a strong capacity to do these things, being a leader will challenge us in ways that we may or may not like.

So, what about those individuals who do have those elements and still cannot lead? Clearly, leadership and the capacity to lead others is complex and requires other abilities. The ability to frame issues in a way that others understand their importance and the necessity to act. The ability to find common ground on solutions. The ability to understand the capacity of others to intervene and a sensitivity to their tolerance for risk.

Much has been written about emotional intelligence and I believe that this capacity is perhaps the most critical aspect of leading. And, as nursing professionals we are often well prepared for the work of emotional intelligence. We learn how to understand the individuals we care for or work with in ways that help us address their needs and to lead them to solutions.

We learn to exchange ideas about what kinds of choices or decisions others make around their health care. We learn to value individuals for who they are and to not judge. All of these are additional essential behaviors for leading others and for full use of our emotional intelligence.

So, leading is action that many nurses have much capacity to fulfill, but many hesitate. Why? Probably because we don't do enough to help nurses learn how to take risks and to understand or experience the rewards of doing that when issues of importance are being addressed. Much of the conversation in this nation about health care—how systems should be designed, what kind of care models should be used, who should deliver certain kinds of service—will not include us as professionals unless we are willing to take risks, assert our authority in these conversations, and lead others to the solutions for better health care.

Leading is risky but it is rewarding. Understanding that you have created solutions by leading others to collaborative work that finds those solutions provides a clear example of how we can fulfill our social mission to improve the health of the public. Without this, we are passive recipients of the environment around us. So, take those risks, challenge your views of how you can or should intervene, and work to lead us forward to a better healthcare world.

REFERENCES

ASHE-ERIC Higher Education Report. (2003). Special issue: Faculty service roles and the scholarship of engagement. *ASHE-ERIC Higher Education Report, 29*(5), 1–161, table of contents.

Balsmeyer, B., Haubrich, K., & Quinn, C. (1996). Defining collegiality within the academic setting. *Journal of Nursing Education, 35*(6), 264–267.

Bass, B. M. (1985). Leadership: Good, better, best. *Organizational Dynamics, 13*(3), 26–40.

Filetti, J. S. (2009). Assessing service in faculty reviews: Mentoring faculty and developing transparency. *Mentoring & Tutoring: Partnership in Learning, 17*(4), 343–352. doi: 10.1080/13611260903284416.

Gard, C. L., Flannigan, P. N., & Cluskey, M. (2004). Program evaluation: An ongoing systematic process. *Nursing Education Perspectives, 25*(4), 176–179.

Green, R. (2005). *Practicing the art of leadership.* (2nd ed.). Upper Saddle River, NJ: Pearson-Prentice Hall.

Haag, P. (2005). Is collegiality code for hating ethnic, racial, and female faculty at tenure time? *Education Digest, 71*(1), 57–62.

Hassna, L., & Raza, S. (2011). An assessment of the relationship between the faculty performance in teaching, scholarly endeavor, and service at Qatar University. *Research in Higher Education Journal, 10,* 1–18.

Jenkins, R. (2006). The service question. *The Chronicle of Higher Education.* Retrieved from Home—The Chronicle of Higher Education chronicle.com/.

Johnston, P. C., Schimmel, T., & O'Hara, H. (2010). Revisiting the AAUP recommendation: Initial validation of a university faculty model of collegiality. *College Quarterly, 13*(2), 1–13.

Kouzes, J., & Posner, B. (2007). *The leadership practices inventory, (LPI).* Retrieved from http://www.leadershipchallenge.com.

Neumann, A., & Terosky, A. (2007). To give and to receive: Recently tenured professors' experiences of service in major research universities. *Journal of Higher Education, 78*(3), 282–310.

Nikou, V. R., In Scheetz, L. J. (2000). Nursing Faculty Secrets, Chapter 7.

Pollicino, E. B. (1996). Faculty Satisfaction with Institutional Support as a Complex Concept: Collegiality, Workload, Autonomy.

Russell, B. C. (2010). Stress in senior faculty careers. *New Directions for Higher Education, 2010*(151), 61–70.

Scheetz, L. (2000). *Nursing faculty secrets.* Philadelphia, PA: Hanley & Belfus.

Story, L., Butts, J. B., Bishop, S. B., Green, L., Johnson, K., & Mattison, H. (2010). Innovative strategies for nursing education program evaluation. *Journal of Nursing Education, 49*(6), 351–354.

ADDITIONAL READINGS

Holling, M. A., & Rodriguez, A. (2006). Negotiating our way through the gates of academe. *Journal of Latinos & Education, 5*(1), 49–64. doi: 10.1207/ s1532771xjle0501_4.

Robert's Rules of Order | Quick Reference. (2012). Retrieved from http:// *www.robertsrules.org/*

CHAPTER 15

The Mentoring Role

CONNIE VANCE

"Imagine classrooms filled with mentor-educators, who having experienced and valuing mentoring, now teach in the framework of affirmation and nurturance of their students in an atmosphere of hope and inspiration—a place where the soil is fertile for healthy growth and change."

—Huang and Lynch (1994) and Vance and Olson (1998)

OBJECTIVES

After reading this chapter, the reader will be able to
- Describe mentoring relationships, roles, and functions
- Understand the value of mentoring relationships for self and others (students and colleagues)
- Describe mentor intelligence
- Know how to create mentor connections and networks for self and others (students and colleagues)
- Understand the challenges and opportunities of mentoring

MENTORING AND MENTORING RELATIONSHIPS

The phenomenon of mentoring is an ancient human activity.

Mentoring is present in every human endeavor—growing up, learning, working, loving, and achieving life's goals and dreams. Whether we realize it or not, each of us has had mentoring involvement in our lives from our families, teachers, co-workers, bosses, and friends. The term "mentor" originally appeared in Homer's Greek myth, *The Odyssey*. In this ancient story, Telemakhos, the young son of King Odysseus, was taught, guided, and protected by Mentor and Athena, the goddess of Wisdom, during the king's

10-year absence fighting the Trojan War. The young prince grew into wisdom and courage through the sustained, caring involvement and influence of his teacher-mentors. In this developmental relationship with the young prince, they served as teacher, coach, advocate, protector, and guide. Mentor and Athena shared their wisdom and experience, promoted Telemakhos' career, and were deeply involved with him personally. "Mentoring is an act of generativity—a process of bringing into existence and passing on a professional legacy" (Johnson & Ridley, 2004, xv). Clearly, the developmental relationship of mentoring is essential to the personal and professional survival, growth, and development of every human being.

In particular, the complexity of nursing and a nursing academic career demands a substantial, ongoing support system and mentor relationships to ensure professional and personal success and satisfaction. Mentoring is an enormously significant component in nursing education. The teaching-learning process—involving teachers, students, and academic and clinical colleagues—is intimately intertwined with mentoring and mentoring relationships. Teaching and learning always occur in relationships with others. Zorn (2010) states that "education is really all three: me (the teacher), the students, and the content. Actually, it is the *relationship* among all three that is education" (p. 21). Some form of mentoring is always present in the teacher-student relationship. Penn, Wilson, and Rosseter (2008) and Bartels (2005) state that an essential skill of the nurse educator is serving as a mentor, role model, and advisor. Mentoring should be present in a teacher's relationships with students inside and outside the classroom and faculty office, in the formal and informal advisement process, and in clinical teaching. Mentoring is also present in various collegial relationships among peers, between junior and senior teachers, clinical partners, and with academic administrators.

The formal mentor-protégé relationship, as illustrated by Mentor/ Athena/Telemakhos, traditionally occurred between an older, more established, experienced person and a younger, less experienced "neophyte." This is very much like the relationship between a teacher and a student, but includes not only the formal academic relationship but the personal as well. This traditional relationship was face-to-face, long-term, exclusive, and intense. However, the mentoring relationship has now evolved to include more breadth and diversity in relation to education, age, experience, background, culture, format, and length of the relationship. We know now that: (1) successful mentoring occurs among peers, as well as between experts and novices; (2) the relationship between mentors and protégés is reciprocal, providing mutual benefits to both protégé and mentor; (3) multiple mentors are more useful than only one exclusive mentor; (4) mentoring can be both formal (assigned) and informal (chosen); (5) mentors can occur in organizational/collective contexts as well as between two individuals; and (6) mentor encounters and networks can be both long-term and of short duration through face-to-face, electronic, telephone, and written vehicles. This broader view is captured in one definition of the mentor connection: a developmental, empowering, nurturing relationship extending over time in which mutual sharing, learning, and growth occur in an atmosphere of trust, respect, and collegiality (Vance & Olson, 1998). This definition reflects the holistic essence and evolutionary nature of mentoring.

MENTOR ROLES AND FUNCTIONS

The academic nurse; i.e., the nurse educator, is engaged in the professional and personal life development and learning of her students, as well as in her own development and learning. Mentoring is at the heart of this developmental process of teaching. In addition, coaching, role modeling, and precepting are aspects of the teacher-mentor's roles and activities. The following encapsulates the meaning of these activities:

Teaching: Imparting knowledge and creating change
Mentoring: Influencing and guiding the career and life.
Coaching: Tutoring and training for specific skills
Role modeling: Providing an ideal for professionalism
Precepting: Orienting and training for the job

Good mentors do many things. Their activities can be broken down into two categories—career functions and psychosocial functions. These, of course, overlap and are complementary. The mentor-teacher will engage in various mentoring activities with their students, depending on the students' needs at different stages of learning and professional development. Teachers themselves will also benefit from expert and peer mentors who provide both career and psychosocial support in the academic setting. The two categories of mentoring assistance are (Vance, 2010):

Career Activities of Mentors	Psychosocial Activities of Mentors
• Guide	• Affirm
• Coach	• Inspire
• Network	• Cheerlead
• Promote	• Counsel
• Open doors	• Support
• Teach	• Advocate
• Model	• Empower
• Protect	• Believe in dreams

THE VALUE OF MENTOR RELATIONSHIPS FOR SELF AND OTHERS

A major goal of the mentor developmental relationship is the promotion of potential, talent, and achievement. Mentors deal in "futures." They believe in the dreams and possibilities of their protégés, hold high expectations of them, and open doors of opportunity. A person can develop and excel without mentoring assistance but the journey is easier, faster, and happier with the presence of good mentors. Whatever the profession or specialty, mentoring is associated with the fuller realization of potential and talent as well as promoting career achievement, satisfaction, and retention of people in that field. Whether one is a neophyte in a new career or a more experienced person who is going back to school or changing a position or career focus (e.g., as a nurse educator from clinical nurse), mentoring is a vital factor in achieving a successful beginning, transition, and ongoing growth and development.

Anecdotal reports and research have consistently demonstrated the benefits of mentoring to all participants in the relationship. Clearly, everyone gains when good mentoring is present. Positive outcomes for teachers, students, nurses, the academic institution, and the nursing profession include (Vance, 2010, p. 36–37):

Enhanced career mobility, success, and achievement
Increased professional, personal, and work satisfaction
Stronger self-confidence and self-esteem
Preparation for leadership roles and activities
Development of talent and potential
Seeking advanced education
Increased motivation and productivity
High performance and excellence in practice
Increased recruitment and retention rates
Empowerment and networking skills
Sustaining a professional legacy

Networks

Mentor relationships are also a key to establishing a strong professional network, which is a cornerstone to your success as a nurse educator. Your network may consist of former and current students, teaching and clinical colleagues, administrators, and friends. Both networking and mentoring entail establishing relationships and connections with others. These mentor networks are important for information sharing; expanding one's knowledge of the academic culture; staying current with trends and issues; developing new skills (e.g., testing and evaluation, grants writing, preparing an academic plan for success); and making new contacts through professional associations and with colleagues who share similar interests. Important networking tools for the nurse educator include the careful development and updating of the curriculum vitae; obtaining a business card from your academic workplace; maintaining electronic and/or paper address books and networking sites, such as LinkedIn; and becoming a member of college and departmental committees and professional associations. The value of mentor networks to your success as a new nurse educator cannot be overemphasized. You will be informed, "connected," and visible to the extent that you are an active networker. Be strategic and creative in finding and expanding networks and mentor connections with administrators, colleagues, and students in many different venues.

MENTOR INTELLIGENCE AND THE NEW NURSE EDUCATOR

Several types of intelligence contribute to achievement and success in a professional role; e.g., the nurse educator. Cognitive intelligence (IQ) and emotional intelligence (EQ) (Goleman, 1995) are two vital ingredients to being knowledgeable and successful in a professional field. A third type of intelligence–mentor intelligence (MQ)–can also provide an enormous advantage in your journey to becoming a nurse educator. Mentor intelligence is the capacity for entering into mentoring relationships (Vance, 2010). It is the ability to *give* and to *receive* mentoring. Mentor intelligence is having the capacity to engage in mentoring your students and colleagues, as well as being open to seek and accept mentoring from others. There are three characteristics of mentor intelligence:

1. Mentoring mentality—*knowing and learning* about mentoring through study, self-reflection, and experience.
2. Mentoring lens—*seeing and viewing* your students, colleagues, and yourself as deserving and needing the benefits of mentoring.
3. Mentoring momentum—*doing and living* mentoring as an attitude and lifestyle in both your mentor and protégé roles.

Mentor intelligence can help you create a culture of mentorship in your relationships with students inside and outside the classroom, in advisement, committee, and professional association meetings, and in clinical areas. MQ can help you create caring educational environments where humanistic teaching and learning relationships occur between teachers and students and among teacher peers and colleagues. MQ cultivates the teacher's compassionate nurturing and guidance of students as they learn professional nursing attitudes, knowledge, and skills. MQ expands leadership growth and opportunities for both your students and yourself in a complex professional and educational journey.

CREATING MENTOR CONNECTIONS AND NETWORKS FOR YOURSELF—THE NOVICE EDUCATOR

Finding good mentors is essential to assist you in developing knowledge and confidence in your role as a novice teacher. The academic culture is different in its values, norms, activities, and language from the clinical culture

(Bellack, 2003). You need a guide and interpreter to help you navigate this new world. In particular, you should seek out expert mentor-colleagues to introduce and guide you in the key academic areas of teaching, scholarship, and service.

The best source of mentors is your faculty colleagues—in both nursing and in other disciplines. These colleagues can share advice, networks, and support about academic life and academic nursing (Vance, 2004). Some academic organizations have created formal mentor programs that match novice teachers with experienced, expert teachers in order to show the novices "the ropes" and direct them through the various avenues of academe. Schools of nursing often create their own distinct mentor programs that address the specific needs of nursing faculty and match seasoned educators with new nurse educators. When a culture of mentorship exists in the school, department, or college/university, individual faculty members also are encouraged to informally seek out their own mentors, and experienced mentors are encouraged to serve as guides to novice teachers. A novice teacher will begin to discover the "stars," experts, and specialists in various fields or disciplines. For example, it is important to know and connect with faculty who are doing scholarly work or research in a particular area. Approaching these colleagues for guidance and involvement is usually welcomed, and is an important entrée to getting one's own scholarship program launched. If a particular colleague is known as a master teacher, it would be wise to ask about attending her classes or seek her advice about your teaching style, methods, and materials.

Another source of mentoring assistance is departmental, school, or college-wide committees. Experienced faculty serve on these committees, and they address agendas integral to the college units and to the faculty. Becoming a member of these committees is an excellent learning resource and mentoring network. As a novice, you will be recognized and appreciated for your service, and you will have the opportunity to access mentors and to expand your network of faculty colleagues.

A particularly important committee to become acquainted with is the college committee that reviews your annual performance and evaluations, and makes recommendations on rank, tenure, and promotion. Nursing programs may have their own committees that begin the evaluation process that is then carried forward at the college level. Nursing faculty usually have a representative on the college-wide rank, tenure, and promotion committee, and you can find guidance from that person, including informational documents related to these aspects of academic life. The college faculty handbook and the nursing program handbook also are essential sources of information for novice nursing faculty.

There is also mentoring help for the new nurse educator through various higher education and nursing education associations. These organizations offer mentoring opportunities through their member networks, workshops, conferences, conventions, journals, websites, Facebook, and various mailings. Some of these organizations have mentor programs for their members to assist them in teaching and faculty-related activities. For nurse educators a great source of mentor networks, educational information, and support are the American Association of Colleges of Nursing (www.aacn.nche.edu), National League for Nursing (www.nln.org), National Student Nursing Association (www.nsna.org), and Sigma Theta Tau International (www.nursingsociety.org) and their school chapters. For example, the American Association of Colleges of Nursing and National League for Nursing have extensive faculty support resources and programs, including materials related to curriculum, teaching strategies and evaluation, faculty and leadership development, funding sources, online courses, networking opportunities, and nursing faculty toolkit. The International Mentoring Association (www.mentoring-association. org) is a broad-based educational and mentoring resource that offers networking, information, and conferences to its members, who are professionals from various disciplines.

Information and networking opportunities also are available through specialty journals, such as *Nurse Educator, Journal of Nursing Education, Journal of Professional Nursing, and The Chronicle of Higher Education. Imprint*, the publication of The National Student Nurses Association, provides a window into the educational resources, leadership opportunities and career guidance for nursing students.

Online mentor networks are increasingly important in higher education for mentoring assistance. These include Education Scholar (www. educationscholar.org), a national health professions program that offers intensive web-based faculty development programs in eight modules; LinkedIn (www.linkedin com), claiming to be the "world's largest professional network"; and *Nursing Spectrum* and Nurse Week (www.nurse.com), that offers educators and students continuing education seminars, webinars, and career advice and networking.

CREATING MENTOR OPPORTUNITIES FOR OTHERS—YOUR STUDENTS AND YOUR COLLEAGUES

As discussed earlier, mentoring is an integral ingredient in the teaching-learning process. Cultivating mentor intelligence will assist you in becoming a significant mentor as part of your teaching role. You will be mentoring your students through your formal and informal relationships with them. You also can be a peer mentor to your academic and clinical colleagues. The teacher who understands the mentor connection and who actively mentors students and colleagues will be a precious scarce resource in academe.

Mentoring Your Students

The first step is to create a culture of mentoring in your classroom, advisement encounters, and clinical teaching. A mentoring culture promotes high-level learning, critical thinking, and professional development—where mutual respect, openness, inquiry, and mutuality of learning and exploration flourish. In mentoring classrooms, shared participative learning occurs between teacher and students and student to student. Participative mentoring learning goes beyond the "lecture-listen" approach. Active participation may include students sharing clinical narratives, collaborating on classroom exercises, using case studies for critical thinking and decision making, and employing both teacher and peer critiques. There are many approaches that a creative mentor-teacher applies in the classroom and clinical settings.

The mentor-teacher also interacts with students in office settings and in college and professional association meetings. Mentoring advisement may include coaching, cheerleading, counseling, role modeling, information sharing, and advocacy—both career-focused and psychosocial-focused activities, as described earlier. Attending college, school, and professional meetings and conferences is another avenue for mentoring and role-modeling professional behaviors, involvements, and advocacy. Students become acquainted with teachers in different contexts and relationships and learn crucial lessons beyond the formal classroom.

Mentoring Your Colleagues

Peer mentoring is a generous gift that helps "grow" the talents of each person in shared learning activities. The give-and-take of exploration and learning with colleagues is exciting and highly productive. It means that we are advocates for each other's contributions and that we showcase the value of nursing and nursing education. Here again, applying mentor intelligence is the key— that we cultivate a mentoring mentality, have a mentoring lens in viewing our colleagues, and create strong support relationships with them. Peer mentoring among colleagues is a priceless resource for the new nurse educator.

THE CHALLENGES OF MENTORSHIP

The enormous benefits of mentoring far outweigh difficulties and challenges. However, because mentor relationships are human relationships, there are potential constraints. To begin with, there may be organizational and professional elements that inhibit the presence and power of mentoring activities. These include authoritarian leadership, workload demands, isolation among colleagues and students, differences in generational and cultural expectations, professional and workplace bullying, scarcity of mentors, lack of collegial trust and sharing, and lack of awareness and knowledge about the need and benefits of mentoring among students and teachers.

There are also potential relational roadblocks that inhibit positive mentoring relationships. Teachers may not see themselves as mentors and prefer to limit their interactions with students in more authoritarian, expert, and disciplinary roles. Students' attitudes toward teachers may come from traditional and authoritarian experiences, and prevent them from reaching out to teachers as potential mentors. Dissimilar backgrounds, values, interests, personality style, role conflicts (i.e., teaching/evaluative versus helping roles), power and control issues, faulty communication, unrealistic expectations, and dependence issues—all of these prohibit open and caring mentor relationships among colleagues and teachers and students.

The greatest barrier of all to developing productive mentor connections is lack of awareness and knowledge about the vital role of mentoring in teaching-learning relationships. The three ingredients of mentor intelligence— mentoring mentality, mentoring lens, and a mentoring momentum—must be cultivated. It is important to be a lifelong student of mentoring, and develop the science and art of mentoring others. "Learn how mentorship works, and practice refining your mentor skills in your daily interactions. Use the word 'mentor' in your thinking and communication with others" (Vance, 2010, p. 146). This requires believing in the power of mentoring, and activating it as a way of thinking and being as a teacher with students and colleagues.

SUMMARY

Our mentor connections as mentor-teachers will affirm and empower each of us, the teaching-learning process, and our profession. The nurse educator is in a pivotal role to influence the practice of nursing for the future by giving and receiving mentoring.

DISCUSSION QUESTIONS

1. Identify two areas in the academic role that you need assistance with. Who could provide mentoring assistance and support in these areas?
2. Discuss how you can raise your mentor intelligence (MQ) in relation to the three components of mentor intelligence.
3. Describe examples of mentoring activities in your teaching, advisement, and professional and personal involvement with students.

SUGGESTED LEARNING ACTIVITIES

1. Develop a self-inventory of your mentor networks to assess the presence and strength of mentoring in your teaching role.
   Include these areas:
   a. Identify key people in your network, why are they important, and list additional persons who should be included in your network.
   b. Identify organizations you belong to, their value to you, and additional groups that could help you in your teaching role.
   c. Describe how you can help students and colleagues build their mentor networks.
2. Make a commitment to nursing's future by giving and receiving the gift of mentoring.

REFERENCES

Bartels, J. (2005). Your career as a nurse educator. *Imprint, 52*(1), 42–44.

Bellack, J. P. (2003). Advice for new (and seasoned) faculty. *Journal of Nursing Education, 42*(9), 383–384.

Goleman, D. (1995). *Emotional intelligence.* New York, NY: Bantam.

Huang, C. A., & Lynch, J. (1994). *Mentoring: The Tao of giving and receiving wisdom.* New York, NY: Harper San Francisco.

Johnson, W. B., & Ridley, C. R. (2004). *The elements of mentoring.* New York, NY: Palgrave Macmillan.

Penn, B., Wilson, L., Rosseter, R. (2008). Transitioning from nursing to a teaching role. *OJIN: The Online Journal of Issues in Nursing, 13*(3), Manuscript 3. Retrieved from www.nursingworld.org/MainMenuCategories/ ANA Marketplace/ANA Periodicals/OJIN/Table of Contents/vol132008/ No3Sept08/NursingPracticetoNursingEducation.Aspx

Vance, C. (2010). *Fast facts for career success in nursing: Making the most of mentoring in a nutshell.* New York, NY: Springer.

Vance, C. (2004). Why teach nursing? *Nursing Spectrum.* Retrieved from http:// include.nurse.com/apps/pbcs.dll/article?AID=2004404050354

Vance, C., & Olson, R. (1998). *The mentor connection in nursing.* New York, NY: Springer.

Zorn, C. R. (2010). *Becoming a nurse educator: Dialogue for an engaging career.* Sudbury, MA: Jones & Bartlett.

PART IV

Scholarly Work

CHAPTER 16

Writing for Publications and Research

"Think and wonder, wonder and think."

—Dr. Seuss

OBJECTIVES

After reading this chapter, the reader will be able to

- Discuss the importance of self-development and shared knowledge
- Understand the significance of publications in refereed journals and tenure and promotion
- Describe strategies for writing for publication
- Identify potential markets for future publications
- Understand the difference between peer-reviewed and non peer-reviewed publications

INTRODUCTION

A spirit of inquiry guides academics in their quest for knowledge. As faculty become more engaged in their roles, they seek to investigate phenomena and expand their knowledge base. This leads them to review current literature, and conduct formal research studies and to share the results through presentations and publications in scholarly journals. Scholarship is an expectation of all faculty but the degree and complexity is influenced by the individual and the expectations of the academic institution. For example, faculty in research-based universities will be required to demonstrate a significant portfolio of research that is funded both internally and externally. Whereas faculty in two- and four-year colleges may be expected to engage in scholarship, it might take the form of collaborative research, scholarly publications, or formal presentations. Thus, some form of scholarship is required for tenure in all institutes of higher education. Scholarship and scholarly work is often equated with research. However, research, albeit one of the highest forms of scholarship, is not the only way to engage in scholarly pursuits.

In fact, faculty must develop a foundational knowledge base and participate in a myriad of scholarly activities before they are ready to conduct formal research. In Chapter 1, an overview of the areas of scholarship that were defined by the AACN and based on the work of Boyer was discussed. The four areas include the scholarship of discovery, scholarship of teaching, scholarship of practice, and the scholarship of integration (American Association of Colleges of Nurses [AACN], 1999).

According to the AACN (1999) the definition of scholarship is:

> Scholarship in nursing can be defined as those activities that systematically advance the teaching, research, and practice of nursing through rigorous inquiry that (1) is significant to the profession, (2) is creative, (3) can be documented, (4) can be replicated or elaborated, and (5) can be peer-reviewed through various methods. (para. 7)

In addition to your own scholarly pursuit you also want to instill in your students a spirit of inquiry by being a role model. This chapter focuses mainly on the scholarship of discovery. As a new nurse educator you will need to decide when the time is right for you to write a scholarly article for a refereed journal, or partake in formal research (Harrison & McKeon, 2010). If you are enrolled in doctoral program, your doctoral dissertation may be your first research project. The following chapter will focus on types of scholarly pursuit.

SELF-DEVELOPMENT

All faculty participate in scholarly endeavors first and foremost to develop themselves as educators and expert teachers. In support of this Robert and Pape (2011) state, "Today, the focus on nursing practice facilitates unity for continued professional development, and is a road to promoting nursing as a recognized and well respected profession. Achievement of this goal was possible through the systematic accumulation of nursing knowledge" (p. 41).

As a new nurse educator you will most likely be entering the field of academia with a strong theoretical and clinical foundation and expertise in a particular field of nursing. This is the foundation that you will continue to develop in addition to learning how to be a master educator. This will require you to spend time reviewing the literature and developing your knowledge in the area of teaching and learning. Additionally, you will continue to expand your knowledge in regard to the content that you will be teaching. So your scholarly pursuit will be focused on the quest for knowledge by participating in conferences and seminars and reading the literature on your subject matter. Additionally you will be engaging in activities that will help you develop your skills as a teacher. You will be learning many new theories and incorporating them into your lessons through the continued development of your courses and teaching content. You will be trying different types of teaching strategies and figuring out which ones work best for you and your students. This should be based on a formal evaluation and measurement of outcomes. You will be learning the art of test development and different ways of evaluation. You will also continue to use student and peer evaluations to guide you through your journey as a nurse educator. During your first year as a new nurse educator a significant amount of your time will be focused on scholarly self-development. Similar to the areas of teaching and service you will want to develop a specific plan on how to meet the expectation of scholarship in regards to continued employment, tenure, and promotion. It is important to check with your academic organization in regards to expectations of scholarly pursuits. Your mentor can also help you to devise a plan that will be realistic. Because many faculty are offered a 9- or 10-month contract they often use their summer months to work on their scholarly endeavors. However, if you are currently enrolled in graduate school you may have to take courses in the summer. Some graduate students are able to write articles related to their course work and their professors can help them with this task. They may even invite students to collaborate on an article with them. Although some academic organizations expect you to write on your own many will accept a co-authored publication. It is a great way to learn the art of writing for publication which is different than the writing you do for your graduate school courses. Although some professors, especially in a doctoral program, will give you assignments that have the potential to be published in a peer-reviewed journal you will have to follow specific submission guidelines of the potential journal.

The National League for Nurses developed the following set of core competencies for nurse educators (Hallstead, 2007):

- Facilitate Learning
- Facilitate Learner Development and Socialization
- Use Assessment and Evaluation Strategies
- Participate in Curriculum Design and Evaluation of Program Outcomes
- Function as a Change Agent and Leader
- Engage in Scholarship
- Function Within the Educational Environment
- Creating an Evidenced-based Practice for Nurse Educators

These competencies may be used as a guide for nurse educators when developing short- and long-term goals. Furthermore, the NLN offers a variety of faculty development courses for new and seasoned nurse educators and a certification test for nurse educators that are based on these competencies. The AACN also offers a variety of faculty development courses for new and seasoned nurse educators. It is important to use a variety of resources throughout your development as a nurse educator.

SHARED KNOWLEDGE

Sharing knowledge is something teachers do on a daily basis. Throughout your career you will be sharing knowledge with your students, colleagues, peers, patients, the nursing profession, and the general public. You will share knowledge on a formal and informal basis. Some ways to share knowledge include teaching, writing for publication, sharing research results, participating in committees, giving presentations, and public speaking. The major way you share knowledge is in your role as a teacher. This is a serious responsibility and you must be sure to utilize the most current and accurate data that is available. As a nurse educator you want to make significant contributions to your profession by engaging in scholarly activities and share the lessons learned with others while serving as a change agent.

TENURE AND PROMOTION

Scholarship influences both tenure and promotion decisions and as you advance up the faculty ranks you will be expected to make significant scholarly contributions. As stated previously teaching is weighed very heavily for beginning nurse educators especially in 2- and 4-year colleges. Engaging in research and publications to advance nursing science is important for all nurse educators even if it is not a major expectation in your academic organization. So how do you know what is expected of you and how do you meet that expectation? Following your organization's policies and the advice of your mentor and dean are you best guides in determining criteria. Some institutions require two or three publications in refereed journals for tenure. Research-based universities will require a track record of research. Most often faculty select a topic they are passionate about and make this their life's work. This often stems from their doctoral dissertation upon which faculty will continue to research and publish on topics related to their body of research.

SCHOLARSHIP AND RESEARCH

Research is most often equated with scholarship and is considered one of the highest and most prestigious forms of scholarly work. The scholarship of discovery includes primary empirical research, historical research, theory development, methodological studies, and philosophical inquiry. Some specific examples include: peer-reviewed publications and presentation of research, theory, or philosophical essays; receiving grants for and positive evaluation of work; mentoring junior colleagues in research and scholarship; and being recognized as a scholar (AACN, 1999). Conducting research is a complex process and as such requires dedication, preparation, and diligence. The coursework you complete in your graduate program should help to prepare you for your future role as a nurse researcher. Before you undertake a research study you need to have an understanding of statistics and types of research. Once you have your topic you need to think about what you are hoping to discover and then select a method of inquiry. Welford, Murphy, and Casey (2011) posit "One of the first requirements when planning research is to establish which paradigm and subsequently which methodology or strategy can best answer the research question" (p. 38). Paradigms in research describe a set of beliefs. They include: "'epistemology' questions the relationship between the knower and what can be known" . . . "'ontology' questions what is the real world and what can be known about it" . . . "'methodology' questions how researchers can go about finding out what they believe can be known" (Denzin and Lincoln (1994), p. 38, as cited in Welford, et al., (2011)). The research paradigms included quantitative, qualitative, and mixed methods. You need to decide what type of study best suits your topic and question. Within both of these types of studies are a variety of methods and methodologies. This is the groundwork for your study. If you choose a quantitative study you will need to decide if it is going to be experimental or non-experimental. You need to be sure to follow all the steps required for the type of research you are conducting. Quantitative research is objective and measurable, and usually involves deductive inquiry, and findings are described statistically. It may be experimental, quasi-experimental, descriptive, or correlational. It is used to test a theory and generate new knowledge. For example, you may decide to investigate patient teaching strategies in young adults who have diabetes. You might compare the use of computer-based instruction and face-to-face instruction to see which method was more effective. Qualitative research is inductive and subjective and the quest for the meaning of life events. Findings are described in themes, concepts, or emerging theories. It includes phenomenology, ethnography, grounded theory, case study research, historical research, philosophical inquiry, and critical social theory. Phenomenological research is conducted to discover the lived experience of the participants; for example, a study on middle-aged adults with multiple sclerosis. Grounded theory is conducted to describe social process such as a healthcare program and data is collected and analyzed until a theory evolves on the issue. Historical research investigates past events and provides a narrative description that can be used to learn about the past and may be used as a foundation for future research. An ethnographic study has its roots in anthropology and is used to investigate and learn about cultures and health practices. In this type of study the researcher becomes immersed in the culture which some describe as "going native" in the field. Philosophical inquiry is an intellectual inquiry relating to foundation or ethical issues in nursing (Burns & Grove, 2009; Polit & Beck, 2012; Welford, Murphy, & Casey, 2011). Critical social theory provides the basis for research on society, communication, and symbols. "Critical nursing science provide a framework from which one may examine how social, political, economic, gender or cultural factors interact to include health or illness experiences" (Ford-Gilboe et al., 1995, as cited in Burns & Grove, 2009, p. 28). After selecting your research question and the type of research study, you will need to follow the specified methodology required for your type of study. You will also need to obtain approval from your Institutional Review Board. You may have an opportunity to collaborate with other faculty in you school or even your clinical partners. Faculty funds may be available but require a formal application process. Be sure to learn as much as possible about the resources that will be available to you throughout your research study. If you have completed a dissertation you should consider conducting another study related to your topic. It is important to be passionate about your topic because you will spend a significant amount of time in this process. After you complete your study, you want to share the results via presentations and publications and should do so as soon as possible because your literature will become dated very quickly.

ADVANCING THE PROFESSION

The profession of nursing is relatively young compared to other professions and it is still developing its own body of knowledge that is based on scientific inquiry. Nurse researchers continue to advance the profession by continuing their education, investigating phenomena through formal reviews and research studies, and by sharing the results with peers and colleagues (Hawranik & Thorpe, 2008). Disseminating results of research studies is vital (Banner, 2011). Many doctoral students spend months or even years conducting their research and completing their dissertation but a good number of them do not try to publish articles from their dissertation. Many scholars note that up to three articles may be written in relation to the dissertation. For example, you might develop an article for a research journal that presents a concise version of your study. Or you might write a review of the literature based on the literature review you conducted for your study. You may also write about the methods you employed for your study or the instruments you used. Another way to advance nursing science is to complete a concept analysis or a review of the literature. You may wish to complete a meta-analysis on quantitative studies, or a meta-synthesis on qualitative studies, or a state of the science paper. Developing and utilizing evidenced-based practice is another way to participate in scholarship especially if part of your role is in the clinical setting (Lehtinen, Öhlén, & Asplund, 2005).

You might also consider writing a policy paper or a clinically based article that presents new or different information. Some journals and magazines invite nurses to write continuing education articles. As you become more experienced you might be asked to contribute to a book by writing a chapter in your area of expertise. However, many experts view writing in peer-reviewed journals as the highest form of scholarship, especially if it is research-based article. Serving as a peer reviewer is a great way to gain insight into the world of publishing and to have an opportunity to review someone's work objectively. You also have an opportunity to add suggestions of important material you think should be included. Writing test items for standardized testing companies is also a great experience and gives you the opportunity to contribute to the profession. When companies are seeking peer reviewers or test item writers they will usually post an open call in their journal or on their website. Of course, there is a formal application and screening process but these roles usually require content experts so look for opportunities in your area of expertise. Initially engaging in scholarly work can be daunting but with experience and support from your mentor and peers you will gain confidence as you embark on your journey as a researcher and a scholar.

GETTING PUBLISHED

The key to getting published is to research the potential journals and their specific submission guidelines and then decide which ones might be best suited for your topic. You need to know what type of articles the magazine publishes. For example, you do not want to send a quantitative research manuscript to a journal that mainly publishes qualitative research. It is very important to read several copies of the potential journal and be sure to follow the writer's guidelines exactly how they are stated. Word count is crucial; manuscripts are rejected all the time because they do not adhere to the required word count. Following guidelines such as APA or MLA and submitting a paper that is well organized, flows well, and has correct grammar and spelling will increase your chances of publication. Bowen (2010) identified seven lessons he learned throughout the process of publishing articles related to his dissertation which was a grounded theory study. Bowen (2010) identified the following seven lessons in publishing qualitative research (p. 865):

1. A dissertation summary won't do

2. Thick description is necessary

3. Collaboration with colleagues has advantages

4. Adherence to guidelines and deadlines is essential

5. "Revise and resubmit" is quite common

6. Electronic journals are not inferior

7. Patience and persistence pay

Although these lessons apply to qualitative research, most of them apply to quantitative research, too. Remember writing is a long and arduous process and it will take many edits and re-writes before you have a well written and polished manuscript. Editors receive hundreds of manuscripts and you have to make yours stand out and be noticed. You need to find a gap in the literature or provide new or unique information on a topic. Always check if a query is required. Some editors prefer a query and will let you know if they are interested in receiving a manuscript on your topic. Of course, there is no guarantee that it will be accepted but you do have a better chance if the editor seems interested. You should always ask a seasoned writer to review your manuscript prior to submission. You want to ask someone who will offer you constructive criticism so you can improve your manuscript. Being published is a lengthy process and it takes a few months to receive a response. The process involves you submitting your manuscript either by snail mail, e-mail, or an online program such as manuscript central. Upon receipt it will be reviewed for compliance with the writer's guidelines and then, if accepted, it will be sent out for a blind peer review by two or three content experts. They will make comments and make a recommendation to the editor. The recommendation may be accept with minor revisions, accept with major revisions, or reject. Although it is disappointing to have a manuscript rejected, do not be discouraged. If you're lucky the editor will include some helpful comments so you can improve your manuscript before you submit it to another market. The important thing is not to give up. If you keep trying and improve your writing skills eventually you will get published.

Even when your article is accepted it will most likely be subject to revisions and edits. You will have to decide if the revisions are acceptable and if so you will need to revise your manuscript and send it back in a timely fashion. There may be several revisions before the final version of your manuscript is approved. Once you have a formal acceptance you may add your publication to your curriculum vitae but instead of the date in parentheses you put (in press). This way you can demonstrate your scholarly work because it may take a year or more before it is actually published. In summary, as a nurse educator in academe you will be expected to engage in scholarly activities. The type and amount of scholarly activity will be dictated by the policies of the academic institution. Engaging in research and writing scholarly articles may pose many challenges but it is well worth the effort. Initially, you may want to collaborate with seasoned faculty members in research and publications until you develop your own expertise.

MARKETS FOR PUBLICATIONS

There are many markets you may consider for your publications. The goal is to find the right niche. To do this you will draw on past experiences and do a thorough review of the market. You should make a list of 10–20 potential markets. If you are in graduate school or finished recently you should be familiar with many of the journals and might want to start with them. You can develop a document or spreadsheet to list the journals, editors, writers' guidelines, page and word count, query requirements, length of review, and whether it is a refereed journal.

You should consider print and online journals. Because of advances in technology and in an effort to be "green," online publications have become quite popular. You will also want to read one or two copies of the magazine to understand the types of articles and style of writing preferred by the editor. Once you complete your list you can consider which one you want to submit to first. As a rule, multiple submissions are not allowed. Another way to search for potential markets is to do a library search or even a Google search. Be sure to check if any of your professional organizations have journals. You might also ask your mentor and faculty colleagues for suggestions. Periodically you should check the various journals for open calls for peer reviewers or specific types of article submissions. A good way to start the writing journey is with an editorial or comments to the editor about an article or topic. Another option is to publish in industry magazines which may not be subject to peer review but will undergo a vigorous review process by the editorial team. This is a great experience and often the editor will give you some wonderful feedback throughout the process. Furthermore, you can add this to your list of publications and although in academia it might not be viewed the same as a refereed article it will still demonstrate your ability to write and be published.

The art of writing for publication requires time, practice, patience, and an ability to accept constructive criticism. You should develop an outline to help you stay focused and organize your thoughts in a logical way. Submitting to a journal or magazine requires you to craft a manuscript that is well organized, and has a good flow, along with clear and concise sentences that make every word count. It is important to delete all unnecessary words. Many new writers become "too attached" to their work and are not able to view it objectively. They may also become upset when an editor wants them to make major revisions. However, the editor is the expert and knows the market. If you want to get published you will have to work closely with the editor. Just keep in mind the mantra "publish or perish" and this will help you to succeed. If you are on a tenure track and hope to advance up the faculty ranks then you will need to publish on a continual basis. Furthermore, as a nurse educator you must try contribute to the profession and advance nursing science. "Despite the importance of this role, nurses have limited confidence and experiences with publishing (Happell, 2005). Interestingly, only 7% of academic nurses publish" (Mcveigh et al., 2002, as cited in Richardson & Carrick-Sen, 2011, p. 756). Richardson and Carrick-Sen (2011) developed an eight-month writing program for nurses in an effort to increase publications. There were 50 participants who attended one or two workshops and by the end of the eight months four participants had been published but 50% of them were still writing. Richardson and Carrick-Sen concluded that the program was valuable but because of time constraints extending the program over one year and helping writers to become more organized with time management would be beneficial. Clearly nurses need continued support and encouragement along the writing journey. In summary, writing for publication may be challenging but with practice, perseverance, and a positive attitude you will be successful.

SUMMARY

This chapter focused on the importance of research and writing for publication to advance nursing science and to earn tenure and promotion. Different types of publications were discussed along with practical advice for getting published.

DISCUSSION QUESTIONS

1. Discuss the four stages of scholarship described by Boyer and adapted by the AACN.
2. Discuss the importance of publication in regard to tenure and promotion.

3. List five strategies for becoming a successful writer.
4. Compare and contrast the difference between peer-reviewed and non peer-reviewed articles.
5. Discuss ways to find potential markets.

SUGGESTED LEARNING ACTIVITIES

▪ Develop a list of five potential markets for publishing your work. You may use the template below or create your own.

Template for Potential Markets

Name of Journal or Magazine	Type of Journal or Magazine	Editor and Contact Information	Submission Guidelines	Preferred Style (APA, MLA, AMA)	Word Count or Page Limit	Query Letter Required	Recent Topics

▪ Write a letter to the editor on a topic or your opinion on a recent article.
▪ Select a journal and write an article based on your area of expertise and the focus of the journal.
▪ Apply to become a peer reviewer for a book, magazine, or journal.

REFERENCES

American Association of Colleges of Nurses. (1999). Defining scholarship for the discipline of nursing. Retrieved from http://www.aacn.org.

Banner, D., & Grant, L. G. (2011). Getting involved in research. *Canadian Journal of Cardiovascular Nursing, 21*(1), 31–39.

Bowen, A. (2010). From qualitative dissertation to quality articles: Seven lesions learned. *The Qualitative Report, 15*(4), 864–879. Retrieved from http://www.nova.edu/ssss/QR/QR15-4/bowen.pdf.

Burns, H., & Grove, S. K. (2009). *The practice of nursing research: Appraisal, synthesis, & generation of evidence* (6th ed.). St. Louis, MO: Saunders/Elsevier.

Denzin NK, Lincoln YS (1994) Handbook of Qualitative Research. First edition. Sage Publications, Thousand Oaks CA.

Ford-Gilboe, M., Campbell, J., Berman, H. (1995) Stories and numbers: coexistence without compromise. *Advances in Nursing Science* 18: 14–26.

Halstead, J. A. (Ed.). (2007). *Nurse educator competencies: Creating an evidence-based practice for nurse educators*. New York: National League for Nursing.

Happell B (2005) Disseminating nursing knowledge—a guide to writing for publication. *Int J Psychiatr Nursing Research 10*(3): 1147–1155.

Harrison, J., & McKeon, F. (2010). Perceptions of beginning teacher educators of their development in research and scholarship: Identifying the "Turning Point" experiences. *Journal of Education for Teaching: International Research and Pedagogy, 36*(1), 19–34.

Hawranik, P., & Thorpe, K. M. (2008). Helping faculty enhance scholarship. *Journal of Continuing Education in Nursing, 39*(4), 155–163.

Lehtinen, U., Öhlén, J., & Asplund, K. (2005). Some remarks on the relevance of basic research in nursing inquiry. *Nursing Philosophy, 6*(1), 43–50. doi:10.1111/j.1466-769X.2004.00197.x.

Mcveigh C, Moyle K, Forrester K, Chaboyer W, Patterson E, St JW (2002) Publication syndicates: in support of nursing scholarship. *J Contin Educ Nurs 33*(2): 63–66.

Polit, D., & Beck, C. (2012). *Nursing research: Generating and assessing evidence for nursing practice* (9th ed.). Philadelphia, PA: Lippincott, Williams, & Wilkins.

Richardson, A., & Carrick-Sen, D. (2011). Writing for publication made easy for nurses: An evaluation. *British Journal of Nursing (BJN), 20*(12), 756–759.

Robert, R. R., & Pape, T. M. (2011). Professional issues. Scholarship in nursing: Not an isolated concept. *MEDSURG Nursing, 20*(1), 41–44.

Welford, C., Murphy, K., & Casey, D. (2011). Demystifying nursing research terminology. Part 1. *Nurse Researcher, 18*(4), 38–43.

CHAPTER 17

Scholarly Activities

"Those that know, do. Those that understand, teach."

—Aristotle

OBJECTIVES

After reading this chapter, the reader will be able to
- Identify types of scholarly activity
- Be knowledgeable about AACN and NLN positions on scholarship
- Discuss ways to engage in scholarly activity
- Understand the importance of joining professional organizations
- Understand the significance of using evidence-based teaching and the scholarship of teaching and learning.

INTRODUCTION

There are many opportunities for nurse educators to participate in scholarly activates.

Nursing is one of the most trusted professions and plays an important role in many organizations. There are multiple conferences locally, nationally, and globally that nurses attend and quite often there are open calls for abstracts for formal oral presentations and poster presentations. Most professional organizations have executive boards or advisory boards and nurse members may be voted into an open position. Nursing organizations are just one of the many other organizations where nurses can play a vital role. The two major professional and accrediting organizations are the American Association of Colleges of Nurses (AACN) and the National League for Nurses (NLN). They both offer a variety of opportunities for professional development and networking. They also both have opportunities for nurse educators to participate in task forces and for experienced nurse educators to fulfill various board membership positions. Your college or university will most likely have a group membership in one or both of these prestigious organizations.

The National League for Nurses (NLN) (2012) identifies the following as the scholarship of teaching:

- Exhibit a spirit of inquiry about teaching and learning, student development, and evaluation methods
- Use evidence-based resources to improve and support teaching
- Develop an area of expertise in the academic nurse educator role
- Share teaching expertise with colleagues and others
- Demonstrate integrity as a scholar

The NLN (2012) identifies the following as scholarly activity:

- Enhance the visibility of nursing and its contribution by providing leadership in the: nursing program; parent institution; community
- Participate in interdisciplinary efforts to address health care and educational needs within the institution; locally
- Promote innovative practices in educational environments

The American Association of Colleges of Nurses (AACN) (1999) identifies the following examples of documentation of the scholarship:

- Peer-reviewed publications of research, case studies, technical applications, or other practice issues;
- Presentations related to practice; consultation reports;
- Reports compiling and analyzing patient or health services outcomes; products, patents, license copyrights;
- Peer reviews of practice;
- Grant awards in support of practice;
- State, regional, national, or international recognition as a master practitioner;
- Professional certifications, degrees, and other specialty credentials;
- Reports of meta-analyses related to practice problems;
- Reports of clinical demonstration projects; and policy papers related to practice.

The AACN and the NLN identify scholarship in multiple areas and these guidelines can be used to determine activities that might be considered scholarship. There are many activities that you can partake in and you should explore all options. During your first year as an educator you may focus on applying for membership in one or two organizations. This will be a good way to start networking and to develop professional association. You will also get to understand the "voice" of the organization and create a list of potential areas for you to become more involved. For example, many organizations seek members to join task forces and to eventually run for a leadership position. Attending one of their annual conferences is a great way to network, and to gain knowledge. You can also see the types of oral and poster presentations that are done by various groups which will help you for your own future presentations. Posters are a good way to start as there is usually a greater number included and it is a more informal type of activity. Developing a specific plan for your scholarly development is highly recommended. It is also beneficial to participate in different types of scholarship which helps you to become more well-rounded and versatile (Pettus, Reifschneider, & Burruss, 2009). All of these activities also help you to develop your role as a teacher as you learn new things and observe other teaching and learning styles by various experts in the field of nursing which you may then apply in your own classrooms (Kalb, 2008). Many experts have defined the term scholar. For example:

> A scholar is an independent thinker who is highly intelligent and takes initiative for pursuing knowledge and for self-learning. This person is honest, generally stands out from the crowd, and yet respects and considers others' ideas, while working to develop new knowledge in the field. (Meleis, 1987; Pape, 2000, as cited in Robert & Pape, 2011, p. 41)

It is sometimes hard to grasp the concept of oneself being considered a scholar but indeed this is a term that is often used to describe nurse educators and researchers. As a new nurse educator you are also on your way to becoming a nurse scholar. Being passionate about something is often the stimulus for many nurse scholars' foray into the pursuit of scholarly development. You have to believe in yourself and seek guidance and help throughout this process. Remember everyone has to start somewhere; scholars are made, not born, so believe in yourself and your ability to succeed.

PROFESSIONAL MEMBERSHIPS

Professional memberships are a requirement for all nurse educators. There are professional organizations for virtually every specialty in nursing so you will have many choices. The key is to join several organizations that relate to your background, expertise, and interests. Most organizations have different levels of membership and require payment of annual dues. Of course, you do have to take into consideration the membership expense so you will have to decide on your budget. Many schools pay for group memberships in the American Association of Colleges of Nurses (AACN) and the National League for Nurses (NLN) so always check with your school to find out membership information. However, if your school does not pay for a group membership you may still join as an individual member. Some organizations are more selective and you must be invited or go through a formal application process to join. For example, Sigma Theta Tau International Honor Society for Nurses invites members based on their academic or leadership achievements. The membership benefits vary based on the organization but most offer online access to resources, networking opportunities, and conferences. They may also have their own magazine or journal and members may have an opportunity to submit a manuscript. Furthermore, there are often annual conferences that you may attend and you may also have an opportunity to submit an abstract for a poster presentation or some type of formal presentation. Professional organizations are a great way to network and you may even have an opportunity to serve on a task force or in a leadership position. The best way to find a potential organization is by consulting with peers and mentors and by conducting a search online for organizations in your area of interest. For example, you may have an interest in critical care nursing and join the American Association of Critical Care Nurses. Or you might be interested in transcultural nursing and join the Transcultural Nursing Society. There are so many options and it may not be feasible to join them all but you should aim for at least three or four organizations that relate to your area of interest. Heinrich, Hurst, Leigh, Oberleitner, and Poirrier (2009) point out that as experienced faculty retire, many of the newer nurse educators are not prepared and lack incentive and time to partake in scholarly endeavors. Furthermore, it was not just new nurse educators who are confused about their role is scholarship and it may take from 10–15 years to become a teacher-scholar. In fact, based on previous studies, Heinrich coined the term *"scholar imposter syndrome"* because many educators held the belief that they could not teach, publish, or conduct research at the same caliber as their the senior researchers and faculty members. This project was developed to offer support and mentorship to emerging faculty scholars. The authors suggest that schools should consider developing orientation and ongoing programs to nurse educators to become teacher-scholars. This is something you should determine as you are seeking your first teaching position. It is important to know what type of support you will have during your transition process and as you work towards tenure and promotion.

PRESENTATIONS

Sharing knowledge through various types of presentations can be an enriching experience for you and the participants who attend your presentation. You may choose to give a presentation with a colleague or small group of colleagues or you may prefer to do it on an individual basis. There are many types of locations and conferences where you might present but you need to seek out these types of opportunities. Posters are a good way to start as there is usually a greater number included and it is more informal process. However, the submission is still competitive and is usually subjected to a peer review. You may decide to develop your own poster or collaborate with someone else. You might also consider sending an abstract for a formal presentation. These are even more competitive and will require development of a PowerPoint presentation and some type of hand-outs. You should consider this in a subject that you are very knowledgeable about and be sure to include the most up-to-date information. Be sure to follow the specific guidelines for topic, format, and word count. If your abstract is accepted you will be required to develop your poster or presentation based on the guidelines and to attend the conference. You might also be asked to participate in a panel discussion in your area of expertise. It is important to note that unless you are an invited speaker you will be required to pay the full amount for the conference, travel, hotel, and expenses so be sure to consider that before submitting. You will want to check with your dean to see if there are funds available to support your attendance at the conference. The cost may be claimed on your taxes as part of your professional role development so you should check with your accountant. You also need to consider your teaching schedule and how you will cover your classes while you are at the conference. You might also try to find conferences that are offered during winter and summer breaks from the school but as long as you develop a plan to address the time you will miss at the college your dean will most likely support your participation. There are many types of conferences that take place, locally, nationally, and globally so you want to explore all options. You might also have an opportunity to present at your school on a topic or if you have recently attended a conference you will be expected to share your experience with your colleagues. It is a good idea to start locally and then expand your sights. There are many civic organizations that invite nurses to speak at community meetings or to volunteer at health fairs. You might even serve as a consultant or speaker at your child's school or your place of worship. These types of activities may be viewed under the umbrella of scholarship and service. Another place to consider is your clinical site. Many hospitals seek nurse educators to give presentations to their staff nurses or to participate in an evidence-based practice study. Or they may have a newsletter to which you can contribute an article in your area of expertise. Malinsky, Dubois, and Jaquest (2010) described the use of institutional ethnography to evaluate programs that also have faculty engage in a scholarly endeavor. They concluded: "Institutional ethnography provided a window into our everyday experiences as nurse educators. While examining our evaluation work, we were simultaneously building our individual and collective capacities to engage in scholarship in various ways, and transforming our teaching practice" (p. 9). This type of activity further demonstrates the wide array of opportunities educators have to engage in scholarship. It is best to have an open mind and think out of the box and you will be surprised at how many ways you can engage in scholarship.

BOARD MEMBERSHIP

Many organizations have different types of boards that often serve in an advisory capacity. Although this was discussed under service, serving as a voluntary member on a board is another way to fulfill the requirement of scholarship. In addition to serving in an advisory capacity, members of boards may also serve on an executive level. As a board member, you need to learn about the organization, review initiatives, and be prepared to offer expert opinions. For example, you may be asked a specific clinical nursing issue or an issue related to nursing education. You might conduct research or a review of the literature on a particular area. Boards are often comprised of members from diverse backgrounds so becoming a member on a board also gives you an opportunity to network and share knowledge. Some examples of boards that seek members are school-based boards, community boards, accrediting and licensing boards, national and international nursing boards, organizational boards, professional and society boards, civic groups, and editorial boards. After serving for several years as a member you may become eligible for a leadership position. Most often this type of position requires a formal election. However, some organizations will invite you to serve in a leadership capacity. You might also be asked to help with grant writing for the various boards you serve on and this is a great experience. If you do accept a leadership position on a board be sure to know exactly what the expectations are and if you will be able to meet them. This type of role often requires regular attendance at meetings which might involve travelling a distance to attend. You may also be required to write reports or participate in a task force. While this is a great experience you must consider if you will have time to accept this type of role. You will also need to know how often your attendance is required and be sure it does not negatively affect your teaching role. Finding a balance is vital and you must be realistic when accepting new roles and responsibilities. Consulting with your mentor and dean can be helpful when making these types of decisions.

SCHOLARSHIP OF TEACHING AND LEARNING

Recently there has been an emphasis in higher education for faculty to demonstrate scholarship and expand knowledge and improve teaching through the scholarship of teaching and learning (SOTL). The scholarship of teaching and learning (SOTL) entails the use of various theories and the continual process of evaluating and improving teaching and learning. Quinnell, Russell, Thompson, Marshall, and Cowley (2010) discuss some of the challenges of sharing knowledge within one's own discipline and with other disciplines. They state, "It is a challenge for academic staff to articulate their narratives about teaching practice in a way that meets the scholarly standards expected in mainstream academic research, either in their own disciplines or as specialists in higher education" (p. 23). Ginsberg and Bernstein (2011) discuss scholarship of teaching and learning (SOTL) in academia. They point out that teaching is the scholarly work that academics engage in and should be considered part of scholarship. However, this is somewhat of a new concept and warrants further investigation and change agents are needed to help their disciplines and their academic organizations embrace this type of scholarly pursuit (Secret, Leisey, Lanning, Polich, & Schaub, 2011).

EVIDENCE-BASED PRACTICE

The use of evidence-based teaching in nursing has become widely embraced and all nurse educators are expected to base their teaching and learning strategies on evidence-based research. It is no longer acceptable to do things because this is the way they have always been done. In academia and in clinical settings research is being conducted to identify best practices based on the evidence. Emerson and Records (2009) define evidence-based teaching in the following way: "Evidence-based teaching practice in nursing is the validation, generation, application, and perpetuation of those methods that facilitate the preparation of skilled and thoughtful nurses who function in a constantly evolving, global health care environment" (p. 361). Thus it is an ongoing process subject to continued review and improvement. Many academics follow the guidelines of the Carnegie Center. "The Carnegie Center for Teaching & Learning is an interdisciplinary resource for the advancement of teaching that emphasizes Boyer's scholarship of application. Its proponents believe that in applying the scholarship of teaching and learning, the learning aspect is essential" (Emerson & Records, 2008, p. 360).

Based on their review of the literature, Emerson and Records (2009) recommend that nurse educators: develop portfolios to demonstrate teaching, scholarship, and service; engage in scholarly discourse with other disciplines; engage in reflection; effectively use resources; and embrace change. As a nurse educator you want to have a spirit of inquiry and base your practice on research and evidence that are related to the scholarship of teaching. That being said you should not be afraid to try new teaching and learning strategies. You just want to develop them based on past and current literature. A pilot study is a great way to test a new type of teaching strategy. For example, you might want to discover the best way to teach nursing students about quality and safety. First you will need to conduct a review of the literature on topics to be included and to discover what types of teaching and learning strategies have been used with positive outcomes. Then you will need to decide your approach. Perhaps you will develop a self-learning module, or a simulation activity, or a written assignment. How will you decide if this is an effective strategy? You might develop a pre-test on the content and a post-test and evaluation tool to be completed after the learning activity. Based on the findings you might revise the strategy or continue to utilize and evaluate to establish reliability and validity. You will want to discuss this with your dean and also determine if you need IRB approval but this type of activity would probably not require IRB approval. More and more educators are being called upon to support their teaching and learning activities with the use of evidence-based teaching and formal evaluation of learning outcomes. Preparing the nurses of tomorrow requires nurse educators who have a continued quest for knowledge and share that knowledge with their students and colleagues. Nurse educators need to be positive role models for their students so that they too will engage in a spirit of inquiry and scholarly pursuit.

SUMMARY

This chapter focused on scholarly activities and the scholarship of teaching. Presenting at conferences and becoming a member of a board or assuming a leadership position were also discussed. An overview of the scholarship of teaching and evidence-based teaching was also presented.

DISCUSSION QUESTIONS

1. Discuss the position of the AACN on scholarship.
2. Discuss the position of the NLN on scholarship.
3. Discuss ways you can engage in scholarly activities.
4. Discuss the benefits of professional memberships.
5. How does the use of evidence-based teaching inform your teaching role?

SUGGESTED LEARNING ACTIVITIES

■ Develop a list of current scholarly activities and develop specific goals for three potential scholarly activities.
■ Identify three to five professional organizations that you might join in the future and investigate the benefits of membership in each one.
■ Select a topic and prepare a mini lesson with a pre- and post-test for evaluation of learning and method of teaching.

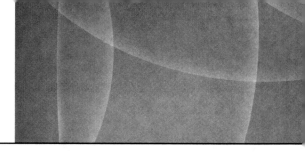

Reflections on Advice for Novice Educators Related to Their Scholarship

TERRY T. FULMER, PhD, RN, FAAN

ONE OF THE MOST IMPORTANT AREAS of development for a new faculty member is the planning, development, and execution of a program of research and scholarship. For those new faculty who are joining a college that is dedicated to a teaching mission, scholarship will take many important forms including expert clinical articles, textbooks, lectures to the community and region and participation in local, state, and national organizations that align with the new faculty member's area of expertise and interest. For those faculty joining research colleges and universities, it is likely that the individual will have completed a post doctoral fellowship and had the benefit of working with a mentor who will have been able to help shape the research and scholarship trajectory in a positive and productive relationship. In most cases, new faculty need to be well versed in the expectations for their research and scholarship productivity before they accept the position.

For new faculty in teaching-intensive colleges, a clear expectation is expertise in teaching and the ability to not only be productive in the classroom, but also to work creatively with syllabi and teaching methodologies which can be seen as a form of scholarship. For example, a nursing faculty member who is expert in geriatric nursing will be able to teach course content in that area but also produce best practice protocols for publication as well as provide commentary on existing protocols and move the practice and teaching forward in that manner. Manuscripts that describe important practice challenges and create strategies for addressing those challenges are essential to the advancement of practice and then the teaching required to educate others around best practices. Protocols related to the state-of-the-art practice expectations around such areas as restraint management, falls prevention, incontinence prevention and management, and pain relief in older adults are all exemplars of how faculty contribute to scholarship while keeping their teaching strategies sharp and current.

In research-intensive universities, it is increasingly the norm that post doctoral fellowships will be highly recommended or required and that a new instructor or assistant professor will join with the plan to get their research underway. Often, the new faculty member will negotiate a reduction in course assignments until some period of time after they have begun their academic appointment. The exact amount of time varies by institution as well as with the new faculty member's level of expertise. It is important that new faculty fully understand the university's expectations before accepting the position to help ensure their academic success.

All new faculty need a mentor. When that mentor is assigned by virtue of a common area of interest between the new faculty and the seasoned mentor, the mentor usually is within the discipline but a preferred "match" may be from other departments in the college or university, depending on the size of the organization and depth of faculty within the same expertise. It is important that new faculty keep in mind that the assignment of the mentor is only a temporary start. If the chemistry between the new faculty and the mentor is not optimal, the new faculty member should request advice on how to shift from the current mentor to a new mentor. The time between the faculty appointment and the very important third-year review goes quickly and it is extremely important that the new faculty member feels comfortable with their mentor and feels that they are getting all the advice and counsel they need to be productive and successful.

It is important to think about lessons learned and I would add a perspective as a former nursing dean and now dean of health sciences. Excellence in teaching is the baseline for staying in the academic setting. Faculty should all be well versed in the pedagogical strategies that are most effective for addressing the content that is to be learned. New faculty often benefit from taking educational seminars related to excellence in teaching skills and they should seek regular feedback from their peers and those individuals to whom they report to ensure that their teaching effectiveness is moving in a steady and positive progression. There will be faculty evaluation forms that are completed by students but further, there should be peer-review evaluations as well as dean evaluations that help guide the new faculty person toward a portfolio that underscores their capacity to be an effective and excellent teacher.

The scholarship and research component of the whole can best be measured by the number and quality of publications in any given academic year as well as important presentations made at professional meetings both regionally and nationally. If new faculty are uncertain as to which of the national meetings are best thought of, they should have that discussion with their dean or chairperson to ensure that they are using their time and resources wisely.

Advice from the directors of research related to small grant initiatives that can help get pilot grants underway is also very important and mentors will be expected to give guidance in this area.

The third part of the tripartite mission in academe is the service component to the institution. Service can take the form of committee work, public service to the community, and service to others. This can take the form of serving as reviewers for manuscripts and grant programs and here again, the advice of a mentor is essential to help the new faculty member sort out work that is productive and important versus work that might be less important.

Transition from any role to the new faculty role needs to be individualized to the person, and new faculty should use their networks to gather the advice and strategy that will put them in the best position for advancement in the academy. Reaching out to senior scholars in the field as well as to scholars in neighboring colleges and universities are all ways that new faculty get good ideas. The caution here is to carefully filter the array and diversity of ideas into a cogent plan that sets you up for success on your journey to promotion and tenure.

REFERENCES

American Association of Colleges of Nurses (1999). Defining scholarship for the discipline of nursing, retrieved from http://www.aacn.org

Emerson, R. J., & Records, K. (2008). Today's challenge, tomorrow's excellence: The practice of evidence-based education. *Journal of Nursing Education*, *47*(8), 359–370.

Ginsberg, S. M., & Bernstein, J. L. (2011). Growing the scholarship of teaching and learning through institutional culture change. *Journal of the Scholarship of Teaching & Learning*, *11*(1), 1–12.

Kalb, K. (2008). Core competencies of nurse educators: Inspiring excellence in nurse educator practice. *Nursing Education Perspectives*, *29*(4), 217–219.

Heinrich, K., Hurst, H., Leigh, G., Oberleitner, M., & Poirrier, G. (2009). The Teacher-Scholar Project: How to help faculty groups develop scholarly skills. *Nursing Education Perspectives*, *30*(3), 181–186.

Malinsky, L., DuBois, R., & Jacquest, D. (2010). Building scholarship capacity and transforming nurse educators' practice through institutional ethnography. *International Journal of Nursing Education Scholarship*, *7*(1), 1. doi:10.2202/ 1548-923X.1948.

Meleis, A. I. (1987). Revisions in knowledge development: A passion for substance. *Scholarly Inquiry for Nursing Practice*, *1*(1), 5–19.

National League for Nurses. (2012). *Certified Nurse Educator (CNE) 2012 Candidate Handbook*. Retrieved from http://www.nln.org

Pape, T. (2000). Boyer's model of scholarly nursing applied to professional development. *Association of periOperative Registered Nurses Journal*, *71*(5), 995–1003.

Pettus, S., Reifschneider, E., & Burruss, N. (2009). Faculty achievement tracking tool. *Journal of Nursing Education, 48*(3), 161–164.

Quinnell, R., Russell, C., Thompson, R., Marshall, N., & Cowley, J. (2010). Evidence-based narratives to reconcile teaching practices in academic disciplines with the scholarship of teaching and learning. *Journal of the Scholarship of Teaching and Learning, 10*(3), 20–30.

Robert, R. R., & Pape, T. M. (2011). Professional Issues. Scholarship in nursing: Not an isolated concept. *MEDSURG Nursing, 20*(1), 41–44.

Secret, M., Leisey, M., Lanning, S., Polich, S., & Schaub, J. (2011). Faculty perceptions of the scholarship of teaching and learning: Definition, activity level and merit considerations at one university. *Journal of the Scholarship of Teaching & Learning, 11*(3), 1–20.

PART V

Special Considerations

CHAPTER 18

Cultural Diversity

"Always remember that you are absolutely unique. Just like everyone else."

—MARGARET MEAD

OBJECTIVES

After reading this chapter, the reader will be able to

- Discuss the importance of teaching a group of culturally diverse learners
- Identify ways to have a positive work experience in a diverse setting
- Discuss issues and strategies related to teaching diverse students
- Discuss the importance of self-assessment and ongoing development
- Discuss issues and strategies related to working with diverse colleagues at the college and clinical settings
- Discuss the importance of including education on transcultural nursing in the curriculum

INTRODUCTION

The age of technology and the World-Wide Web have facilitated the globalization of our world. Today most classrooms and workplace settings are comprised of people from many different backgrounds and lived experiences. Some of the most common differences relate to culture, ethnicity, religion, gender, and age. However, as cultures become entwined, subcultures emerge so it is important not to compartmentalize or stereotype based on any one particular group (Buscemi, 2011). The culturally diverse classroom is one that is both educationally stimulating and at times challenging. Identifying one's own personal beliefs and learning about the various cultures is recommended for all nurses and a requirement for all educators. Because we live in a global society that is constantly changing, learning about the uniqueness of the various cultures and subcultures is actually a lifelong process. Culture will impact your role as an educator, colleague, and care giver. Not only do you need to become culturally competent, you also need to mentor your students in understanding and applying concepts of cultural care in the classroom and clinical setting. In this chapter, an overview of various cultures and ways to address the unique learning needs of a diverse group of students will be presented.

CULTURE

Culture is a word that describes many facets of daily living. According to the Merriam-Webster dictionary culture is "the customary beliefs, social forms, and material traits of a racial, religious, or social group; *also*: the characteristic features of everyday existence (as diversions or a way of life) shared by people in a place or time" (Merriam-Webster, 2012). A person's culture and cultural beliefs influence virtually every part of their life. In the workplace employees need to respect one another and try to understand one another's beliefs. As an educator you need to understand how a student's culture affects his/her behavior and their unique learning needs (Campesino, 2008). As a nursing educator you will also be teaching students how to provide culturally congruent care to a diverse group of patients. You will serve as a role model for students by demonstrating collegiality in the workplace and cultural sensitivity in the classroom. Completing a self-assessment of your cultural values, beliefs, and attitudes is the first step in developing cultural awareness (Jeffreys, 2010). Developing a knowledge base of various cultural beliefs and practices that you continue to build upon is the next step. Taking that knowledge and incorporating it into your classroom and workplace are equally important.

CULTURAL AWARENESS

Learning about different cultures will help you in your workplace and in the classroom. Although it is not possible to know all cultures, having a basic understanding of some of the predominant cultures in your geographic location is helpful. As you develop as an educator you will be expanding your knowledge base on the various cultures. This knowledge will inform your role as a peer, mentor, colleague, and teacher. Schriner (2007) conducted a qualitative study on the relationship of culture and transition of new faculty and found that there is a dissonance between new faculty beliefs and expectations and the academic setting. She posits that cultural change is needed so that values and beliefs are shared between the institution and the faculty. Every organization has its own culture and new faculty need time to learn this culture. Organizations should provide a thorough orientation and a mentor to help new employees learn the expectations and culture of the organization and its members. Learning about various cultures gives one an understanding of values, beliefs, and practices. Although one might not always agree with these practices it is important to respect each person's individuality. To help you on your cultural journey an overview of several cultures will be presented in the following section. This may serve as a review for some and for others may be new information.

African Americans are the third largest population in America and according the U.S. Census Bureau (2010) the black population is 12.6%. This population includes people from Africa, South and Central America, and the Caribbean, many of whose ancestors were originally brought here as slaves. The African American culture has values and beliefs that have been influenced by their original country of origin and the American European culture (Scott, 2005).

African Americans have several different religious beliefs. According to Purnell (2009) a large number of African Americans belongs to Methodist or Baptist churches. However, other religions embraced by traditional African religion-Americans include Jehovah Witness, Roman Catholic, Islam, and African. Because of the influence of subcultures there are some rituals that are embraced by this population irrespective of their religious affiliation, such as the laying on of hands for healing and keeping the body intact after death. The predominant language is English but they may use particular words and phrases that are unique to their culture. Some birth rituals include not taking pictures of the pregnant women which may result in stillborn births, food cravings, not raising arms above the head, and taking castor oil to induce labor. Eye contact is acceptable but if prolonged may be considered confrontational. Respect is very important and most people prefer to be called by their surnames. African Americans place a high value on education. However, due to economic issues they may not be able to help all their children with college tuition so they strive to have at least one of their children earn a college degree.

The Hispanic or Latino population is approximately 16% of the total population in America (U.S. Census Bureau, 2010). This population includes people from Mexico, Central and South America, Puerto Rico, Cuba, and the Dominican Republic. Hispanic is not a culture; it is actually a classification that was developed in the 1970s by the U.S. Census Bureau to classify people that were connected by Spanish language or culture. Because the Hispanic population is comprised of so many people from different cultures there are very distinct differences based on country or island of origin. It is important not to stereotype. However, there are some common beliefs and values that are applicable to many Hispanics. Marriage and family are extremely important to this culture and Catholicism is the predominant religion. Family and respect, especially for parents and elders, are very important. Eye contact, while acceptable is dictated by age, sex, position, and authority; eyes are kept downcast to show respect. Many decisions are made by the family as a whole and when important events take place the entire family will attend. Some Hispanics believe in "mal ojo" (evil eye) which may cause illness such as vomiting and may require the intervention of a curandero to heal the person. They may also believe in "hot and cold" diseases that are treated with the opposite temperature. For example, since pregnancy is considered a "hot" condition cool or cold types of foods and temperatures are recommended. Pneumonia is considered a "cold disease" so hot temperatures and foods such as teas and soup would be recommended. They also use many different types of herbal remedies for healing (Andrews & Boyle, 2008; Galanti, 2008; Purnell, 2007).

Asian-Americans comprise about 4% of the population in America and include people from China, Japan, Korea, India, and the Philippines. Language and religious beliefs varies based on country of origin. For example, many people from the Philippines are Catholic; while others practice Buddhism, Hinduism, or the Muslim religion. Education is of high important to Asian-Americans. Eye contact can be viewed as disrespectful or aggressive and therefore it is common for Asian people to keep eyes downcast when communicating. A greeting with a bow or handshake is generally acceptable. They are very respectful of their elders and people in authority. They strive for balance between Ying and Yang. They may follow Western medicine but believe in many Eastern healing practices such as acupuncture, meditation, herbs, and teas. The Native Americans which include American Indians and Alaskan Natives, comprise approximately 0.9% of the total population. There are over 500 tribal governments that are recognized by the United States. These individual tribes govern their reservations and people, and cultural beliefs and practices vary among tribes. Today many Native-Americans live on reservations. They are often quiet and use silence as a way to show they are listening and usually keep eyes downcast to show respect. They are very respectful of nature and although they may accept Western medicine practices they also belief in balance and harmony. They may use shamans (healers), herbal medicine and teas, rituals, dances, chanting, and body painting to treat illnesses which many believe is caused by spirits. Arab-Americans comprise approximately 0.5% of the total population in America and include people from the various Middle Eastern countries, such as Lebanon, Palestine, Egypt, and Libya. Many of them are Muslim and still adhere to their strict beliefs of modesty (women dress in traditional clothing), religious practices, and dietary restrictions. Caucasians are the largest group in the United States and according to the census bureau comprise 72.4% of the total population. This population includes people from North America, Europe, Africa, and Australia. Ethnic groups in the white population include German, English, Irish, Italian, Polish, Russian, Greek, and French. Because many of these groups have been here for a long time their cultural beliefs and practices are a combination of their heritage and the American culture. They most often subscribe to Western medicine and more traditional beliefs. However, many also embrace some type of Eastern medicine such as meditation and herbal remedies. Religious beliefs vary based on country of origin and include Catholicism, Judaism, and Christianity. Celebrations include American holidays and cultural ones. Eye contact and hand shaking are norms and considered a sign of respect.

When considering culture one must take into consideration many factors and be careful not to stereotype. People are constantly changing and will usually identify with different subcultures. Within each main culture are variations based on a variety of factors. For example, the longer you live in an area you may become acculturated and adopt some of the values, beliefs, and practices that are unique to that culture. Specific families have their own subculture. Organizations, schools, and classrooms have a unique set of cultural values, beliefs, and practices that are influenced by the past and present populations. It is important to note that organizational culture is continually evolving as new members join and bring their unique set of values, beliefs, and practices. Furthermore, within organizations are many different subcultures which relate to ethnicity, religious beliefs, gender, age, and role.

THE CULTURALLY DIVERSE CLASSROOM

The typical classroom of today, especially in colleges and universities, is usually comprised of a very diverse group of learners. Because of this it is important to consider how cultural beliefs and practices influence learning. Communication in the form of verbal, non-verbal, and written word may cause misunderstandings and issues with students and faculty. Because different words and gestures may have different meanings to different groups of people one must carefully select one's verbiage. Furthermore, students who did not receive their primary education in this country or whose native language is not English may have difficulty with taking multiple-choice tests or writing scholarly papers. Faculty need to help these students to get the support they need through the various academic support programs at the college or university (Jeffreys, 2012). Being sensitive to behaviors that demonstrate respect such as eye contact, personal space (proxemics), touch, and tone of voice will help to create a positive learning environment for all. Beyer (2010) posits that most teachers feel they are not adequately prepared to teach in a multicultural classroom. Furthermore, she posits that three areas have been identified to address this issue: "These goals include teaching stakeholders in schools to appreciate diversity and accept pluralism, reduce prejudice, and infuse the curriculum with multicultural materials and concepts" (p. 120). As a nurse educator you want to serve as a role model for your students and peers. You also need to advocate for your students and identify strategies that will help them feel a spirit of inclusiveness. Being aware of your verbal and non-verbal communication and how words or gestures may be misunderstood is vital. Personal space must be considered as some people do not feel comfortable if someone gets too close. Touch is also best avoided as some cultures do not feel that touching is appropriate. Eye contact must also be considered. Sometimes words and gestures have different meanings in different cultures so it's important to be very clear when communicating. Words may have different meanings or connotations in different countries. "In Mexico the word *horito* means right now. In Puerto Rico the same word means in an hour or so" (Galanti, 2008, p. 28). Gestures may also be misinterpreted; for example, the "okay" sign that people make with their thumb and pointer finger means "everything is okay or good" in America. However, in Japan this sign means "money" and in France it is considered a "zero" so a person may think you are telling them they are "worthless." The "thumbs-up" gesture is something positive in America, but is a curse word in Greece and means the number one in most European countries. You can imagine how a Greek student might feel if they give a correct answer and as the teacher you respond with the thumbs-up sign. It is best to avoid these types of gestures but if you do use them in a diverse setting then you should explain their intended meaning. Furthermore, it is best to avoid idioms and slang words, especially with ESL (English as second language) students because their interpretation of words is usually more literal. It is a good idea to let students know at the beginning of the semester that they should always ask for clarification. Although some students, especially Japanese, may not feel comfortable telling you they do not understand in order to "save face" they may just nod in agreement. Another issue that needs to be clarified is time orientation because in America punctuality is very important. Some cultures do not put as much emphasis on punctuality so it is important to be clear about this expectation (Andrews & Boyle, 2008, Galanti, 2008; Jeffreys, 2010; Purnell, 2007). To help faculty address the needs of diverse learners Jeffreys (2010) developed the DIVERSE acronym to guide teachers (see Figure 18.1).

FIGURE 18.1

Acronym for Meeting the Needs of Diverse Learners

Plan for Meeting Needs of Diverse Learners	
Developmental	A developmental approach is recommended whereby a comprehensive, broad introduction to cultural competence and transcultural nursing provides a foundation for subsequent cultural competence education. Subsequent teaching-learning strategies purposefully weave together and build upon prior formalized and informal learning in order to foster optimal cultural competence development. The developmental approach integrates cognitive, practical, and affective learning at increasingly higher levels throughout the educational process.
Immediate	Immediate relevance and direct application into the clinical or work setting is consistent with adult learning theory that recognizes the uniqueness of adult learner populations.
Variety	A wide variety of learner-centered teaching-learning activities partnered with a wide variety of case study examples representing a wide variety of cultural groups and clinical needs is recommended for the wide variety of academically and culturally diverse health care professionals and students requiring ongoing cultural competence education.
Evidence-based	Empirically supported teaching-learning strategies should begin the repertoire of teaching-learning strategies implemented and evaluated in academic, health care, and professional association settings. Adaptation of existing strategies and the design of new teaching-learning strategies should be routinely appraised for the achievement of successful outcomes. Both formative and summative evaluations, routinely conducted, will add to the repertoire of evidence-based teaching learning strategies

(continued)

FIGURE 18.1 Acronym for Meeting the Needs of Diverse Learners (*continued*)

Plan for Meeting Needs of Diverse Learners	
	most effective in cultural competence education. Evaluating what strategies work best for various sub-groups of diverse learner will be instrumental in meeting the needs of diverse learners and enhancing optimal cultural competence education.
Resources	Pooling together appropriate human, financial, scholarly, and space/equipment resources will maximize opportunities for a positive learning experience and enhance optimal cultural competence development. Without sufficient resources, cultural competence education will be adversely affected.
Selective	Selective case scenarios and learning experiences should be guided by pre-determined priority needs of learners or key targeted patient groups (clinical setting) or students (academic or continuing education setting).
Experiential	Guided and mentored experiential learning experiences, preceded by key preparatory learning activities, provide a tremendous opportunity for developing optimal cultural competence. Actual performance of transcultural nursing skills or culturally specific actions is most influential in transcultural self-efficacy appraisal and the further development of cultural competence knowledge, skills, and attitudes, and confidence.

From Jeffreys, M. (2010). *Teaching cultural competence in nursing and health care: Inquiry, action, and innovation* (2nd ed., p. 128). Reprinted with permission of Springer Publishing Company, New York, NY.

RELATIONSHIPS

Creating a culturally congruent classroom requires collaboration between faculty and students. It is helpful to try to view your curriculum, syllabus, content, lesson plans, books, references, and exams through the eyes of your diverse students. For example, how would you feel if you were the only student who was different? Or if you did not have a good command of the language spoken? Or if all the books and videos were based on one culture that was quite different from yours? It is important to select books and other material that is representative of various cultures. PowerPoints and other audio-visual aids should be culturally diverse. A great way to help students feel more comfortable and to recognize different cultures is to have cultural celebrations where faculty and students bring in ethnic foods and share information about their culture. Because becoming culturally congruent is a process you should conduct frequent self-reflection, and evaluation of curriculum, lesson plans, and learning outcomes should be done on a continual basis (Quaye & Harper, 2007). Jeffreys (2010), who has written extensively on cultural competence in nursing, has developed the acronym HOLISTIC COMPETENCE for faculty (Figure 18.2).

FIGURE 18.2
HOLISTIC COMPETENCE Acronym

<u>H</u>uman-connectedness	between faculty and students makes a powerful difference in retention
<u>O</u>ptimization	focuses on enrichment for everyone to achieve maximum potential
<u>L</u>earner-centered	strategies engage learners in immediate professional application and relevance
<u>I</u>ndividualized	strengths and weaknesses of diverse students must be addressed
<u>S</u>cientifically-based	retention strategies provide a beginning repertoire of ideas and data
<u>T</u>eamwork	must be emphasized at all levels (faculty, staff, administration, students)
<u>I</u>ntegrated	retention efforts must be carefully woven throughout the organizational fabric
<u>C</u>reative	ideas and innovations must address academic and nonacademic issues
<u>C</u>aring	sincerely about holistic needs of students is the first step in fostering success
<u>O</u>ngoing	and coordinated retention interventions throughout the program is essential
<u>M</u>ultidimensional	strategies must correspond with multidimensional factors influencing retention
<u>P</u>roactive	strategies are initiated before problems occur and at key transitional periods
<u>E</u>thics	and accountability underscore the need for full faculty involvement
<u>T</u>rust	is an essential component for building an open, caring learning environment

(continued)

FIGURE 18.2 HOLISTIC COMPETENCE Acronym (*continued*)

Education	for meeting the holistic needs of students includes formal & informal forums
Networks	with experts and others on best practices for student retention expands ideas
Confidence	influences student commitment, motivation, and persistence behaviors
Evaluation	of strategies implemented provide guidance for future innovations

From Jeffreys, M. (2012). *Nursing student retention: Understanding the process and making a difference* (2nd ed., p. 128). Reprinted with permission of Springer Publishing Company, New York, NY.

THE CULTURALLY DIVERSE WORKPLACE

Many of the cultural issues to consider in the workplace are similar to the strategies utilized in the classroom. Collegial relationships, communication, and respect should be the common goal of all the members of the organization (Maier-Lorentz, 2008). Sreedar states "For a wide assortment of employees to function effectively as an organization, human resource professionals need to deal effectively with issues such as communication, adaptability and change" (2011, p. 34). Most organizations recognize the importance of cultural diversity and have programs and policies in place. However, there is often a dominant culture in an organization and many employees expect that new employees will assimilate to this dominant culture. Organizations have to be fully committed to embracing cultural diversity. Barriers to cultural diversity include stereotyping and prejudice. Many people have preconceived opinions about a particular group or culture and may be very rigid in their views. Leaders should be role models and develop policies and programs that will foster a sense of collegiality (Lopez-Rocha, 2006). As a nurse educator you will be addressing culture in several ways. First and foremost you will be creating a spirit of inclusiveness in your classroom while continuing to learn about the various cultures, values, and beliefs of your students. You will also need to learn the culture of your organization as a whole and the culture of your particular school or department. If one of your roles is to teach clinical, you will need to learn the culture of your clinical site. Hospitals must demonstrate compliance with the Joint Commission on all of its standards which includes cultural competence. Even though you are not an employee of the clinical site where you teach, you and your students are still expected to comply with all standards, policies, and procedures. You will want to serve as a role model for your students by understanding and applying concepts on culturally congruent care.

TRANSCULTURAL NURSING

Leininger is considered the foundress of transcultural nursing. She developed the Culture Care Theory (1978) based on her research as a nurse anthropologist. "Transcultural nursing is a specialty within nursing focused on the comparative study and analysis of different cultures and subcultures" (Andrews & Boyle, 2008, p. 4). "The *purpose* and *goal* of the theory is to use research findings to provide culturally congruent, safe, and meaningful care to clients of diverse or similar cultures" (Leininger, 2002, p 190). The overall goal is to continue to develop a body of knowledge that is focused on the relationship of culture to health and illness and for nurses to provide holistic care that is culturally congruent. Dr. Leininger developed the Sunrise Enabler Model (see Figure 18.3) to help nurses understand the concepts of culture care and to base their holistic nursing care on the various parts of the model. "All data from the top and middle of the Sunrise Model are reflected on with the three modes of decisions and actions to arrive at culturally congruent care (bottom part of model)" (Leininger, 2002, p. 192). This model demonstrates how important holistic nursing care is to all patients. It also helps nurses to understand the importance of considering many factors when providing culturally congruent care. Today most schools of nursing teach transcultural nursing to their students. Some schools have specific courses and others integrate the concepts and theories throughout the curriculum.

Jeffreys (2010) points out that culturally congruent care is a patient's right and has legal and ethical implications. Furthermore, there is evidence that supports the positive effect of culturally congruent nursing care on patient outcomes. Nurse educators are responsible for teaching their students about cultural caring and should serve as role models. There are a plethora of resources and many opportunities for "teachable moments" in theory and clinical courses. One caveat is to be sure that students understand that they should be careful not to categorize patients based on their backgrounds. The individual needs of the patient should always be considered because everyone is unique and within each dominant culture are many different subcultures.

A more recent model was developed by Purnell and Paulanka (1998) called The Purnell Model of Cultural Competence. According to Purnell (2002) "A culturally competent health care provider develops an awareness of his or her existence, sensations, thoughts, and environment without letting these factors have an undue effect on those for whom care is provided" (p. 193). Purnell's model has 12 domains that are depicted in a circle with global society being the outer ring followed by community, family, and person. This is followed by 12 wedges with the domains that have cultural concepts that are all utilized to inform culturally congruent care. The 12 domains in this model are (Purnell, 2002):

- Overview/heritage
- Communication
- Family roles and organization
- Workforce issues
- Biocultural equality

FIGURE 18.3
Leininger's Sunrise Enabler to Discover Culture Care. Reprinted with
permission from Leininger (1995).

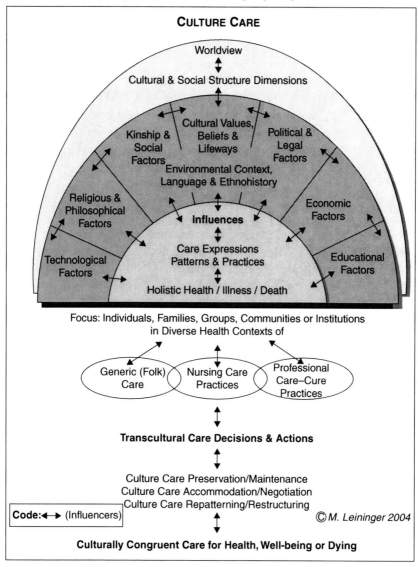

- High-risk behavior
- Nutrition
- Pregnancy and childbearing practices
- Death rituals
- Spirituality
- Health care practice
- Health care practitioner

All of the domains are related to one another and influence each other. They are representative of the areas health care practitioners need to consider when providing culturally congruent care. Utilizing models can help health care practitioners to properly assess and provide care that is based on the unique needs of the individual.

SUMMARY

This chapter focused on the different aspects of culture in relation to the workplace, classroom, and health care setting. An overview of several cultures was presented along with strategies for providing culturally congruent care.

DISCUSSION QUESTIONS

1. What is the difference between a culture and a subculture?
2. Discuss the issue of eye contact and its significance in different cultures.
3. What is the difference between stereotyping and prejudice?
4. Discuss strategies for effective communication with diverse groups.
5. Compare and contrast Leininger's Model of Culture Care and Purnell's Model of Cultural Competence.

SUGGESTED LEARNING ACTIVITIES

▪ Develop a course offering for a diverse group of learners utilizing culturally sensitive teaching and learning strategies.
▪ Interview the HR director at a local hospital about their cultural competency program.
▪ Attend a cultural event or cultural museum and write an essay about the experience
▪ Interview two faculty members on how culture affects their teaching.

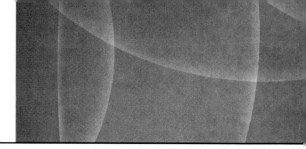

Diverse Learners

MARIANNE R. JEFFREYS, EdD, RN

I FEEL AN ENERGIZED ANTICIPATION WHEN teaching diverse learners. It is an unbelievable opportunity! I feel both humbled and privileged to work with diverse learner populations at various stages of career development beginning with pre-nursing advisement, associate degree, RN-BS, master's, through doctoral degrees. How thrilling it is to meet a baccalaureate or master's level class for the first time and discover one student or several whom I remember from 3 years, 5 years, or even 20+ years before during their first fundamentals of nursing course! Some of these students had been at-risk for dropping out or failing out or giving up. Yet they were now transformed into nursing professionals, providing valuable services to diverse patients, and moving forward in their careers. How wonderful! It also felt wonderful when many former students thanked me for linking them with a peer mentor-tutor (PMT), organizing PMT-led study groups, and creating a multiservice Nursing Student Resource Center, noting that their formal and informal interaction with diverse role models motivated them to persist and strive towards realistic goals previously inconceivable.

Sparking inquisitive curiosity, igniting passion for the nursing profession, nurturing realistic self-efficacy (confidence), and fostering the belief in one's valuable contributions to nursing and health care among my diverse learners necessitates focus on my own learning—about new strategies and techniques to uncover the potential within diverse learners so that their passion and creativity may emerge, flourish, and inspire others. All too often, students (especially beginning nursing students), hold unrealistic expectations—either inefficacious or overly confident. Both are dangerous in jeopardizing successful outcomes.

*What **can** we do?* Discover the motivational forces deep within, capitalize on student strengths, pair students with similar and different strengths and weaknesses to encourage dialogue, and a true, sincere joy in others' successes becomes a shared celebration for all.

*What else **must** we do?*

▨ Embrace the diversity of diversity. Doing so fosters one's own ongoing development as a person and as a nurse educator.
▨ Don't allow the fear of mistake or failure or the unknown deter you from embarking on a whirlwind, exhilarating journey of life and nurse educator. The privilege of preparing future generations of nurses for a compendium of current and future possibilities and interprofessional roles locally, nationally, globally, and interplanetarily, requires an out-of-the box approach that begins with embracing the diversity of diversity.
▨ View diversity as a strength. Diversity exists in many forms such as birthplace, socioeconomic status, age, gender, primary language, monolingual or multilingual, neighborhood, sexual orientation, religion, ethnicity, national origin, politics, etc.
▨ Appreciate the various viewpoints and perspectives and life experiences that a diverse learner group brings to a formal or informal learning setting.
▨ Be open to new ideas but don't be myopic in seeing only differences; look for the similarities that connect differences towards a mutual goal. The goal of providing high quality, culturally competent health care to individuals, families, and communities around the world and beyond by preparing diverse nurses and learners who are happy, motivated, and appropriately challenged to go beyond complacency and the status quo demands that nurses question and be visionary, think outside the box, and propose innovative, creative solutions to new and old problems.

The opportunity to continually learn from my students and interdisciplinary colleagues instills a renewed quest to implement cutting-edge evidence-based strategies for diverse learners and to propose and test new ideas and innovations for future generations of learners and nurse educators. The future can either unfold or the future can be shaped by open-minded, creative, visionary, committed, dedicated nurse educators who ignite every learner's passion to contribute uniquely to the nursing profession and health care. Let's join together in shaping the future of nursing by capitalizing on the unique qualities that diverse learners and educators bring to the profession and society!

REFERENCES

Buscemi, C. P. (2011). Acculturation: State of the science in nursing. *Journal of Cultural Diversity, 18*(2), 39–42.

Andrews, M., & Boyle, J. (2008). *Transcultural concepts in nursing care* (5th ed.). Philadelphia, PA: Wolters Kluwer & Lippincott.

Beyer, C. (2010). Innovative strategies that work with nondiverse teachers for diverse classrooms. *Journal of Research in Innovative Teaching, 3*(1), 119–129.

Campesino, M. (2008). Beyond transculturalism: Critiques of cultural education in nursing. *Journal of Nursing Education, 47*(7), 298–304.

Galanti, G. A. (2008). *Caring for patients from different cultures* (4th ed.). Philadelphia, PA: University of Pennsylvania Press.

Jeffreys, M. (2010). *Teaching cultural competence in nursing and health care: Inquiry, action, and innovation* (2nd ed.). New York, NY: Springer Publishing Company.

Jeffreys, M. (2012). *Nursing student retention: Understanding the process and making a difference* (2nd ed.). New York, NY: Springer Publishing Company.

Leininger, M. (1978). *Transcultural nursing.* Thorofare, NJ: Slack.

Leininger, M. (1995). *Transcultural nursing: Concepts, theories, research, and practices.* Columbus, OH: McGraw-Hill.

Leininger, M. (2002). Culture care theory: A major contribution to advance transcultural nursing knowledge and practices. *Journal of Transcultural Nursing, 13,* 189–192.

Lopez-Rocha, S. (2006). Diversity in the workplace. *International Journal of Diversity in Organisations, Communities & Nations, 5*(5), 11–18.

Maier-Lorentz, M. (2008). Transcultural nursing: Its importance in nursing practice. *Journal of Cultural Diversity, 15*(1), 37–43.

Merriam-Webster Online Dictionary. (2012). Retrieved from http://merriamwebster. org

Purnell, L. (2002). The Purnell model for cultural competence. *Journal of Transcultural Nursing, 13*(3), 193–196.

Purnell, L. (2009). *Guide to culturally competent health care* (2nd ed.). Philadelphia, PA: F. A. Davis.

Purnell, L., & Paulanka, B. (1998). *Transcultural health care: A culturally competent approach.* Philadelphia, PA: F. A. Davis.

Quaye, S. J., & Harper, S. R. (2007). Faculty accountability for culturally inclusive pedagogy and curricula. *Liberal Education.* p. 32.

Schriner, C. L. (2007). The influence of culture on clinical nurses transitioning into the faculty role. *Nursing Education Perspectives, 28*(3), 145–149.

Scott, H. (2005). *The African-American culture. Viewpoint commentaries on the quest to improve the life chances and the educational lot of African Americans.* Retrieved from www.pace.edu/.../VP-THEAFRICANAMERICAN CULTURE_Hugh_

Sreedhar, U. (2011). Workforce diversity and HR challenges. *Advances in Management, 4*(10), 33–36.

USA QuickFacts from the US Census Bureau. (2010). Retrieved from http:// quickfacts.census.gov/qfd/states/00000.html

CHAPTER 19

Students With Disabilities

"A pessimist sees the difficulty in every opportunity; an optimist sees the opportunity in every difficulty."

—Sir Winston Churchill

OBJECTIVES

After reading this chapter, the reader will be able to

- Discuss the legal issues relating to educating nursing students with disabilities
- Understand the significance of the legal issues addressing students with disabilities
- Discuss faculty responsibility in educating nursing students with disabilities
- Discuss student responsibility relating to admission, self-disclosure, and accommodations and learning disabilities

INTRODUCTION

All students face multiple challenges in the educational setting, and for students with disabilities these challenges are magnified. Nursing students with disabilities may require additional strategies and accommodations to be successful. The Americans with Disabilities Act (ADA) was developed to protect the rights of people with disabilities. It was originally created in 1973 as the Rehabilitation Act and went through several revisions and endorsements. In 1990 the Rehabilitation Act of 1973 was amended to reflect the principles of the ADA which resulted in the American Disabilities Act and Section 504 being signed into law in July of 1990. The most recent endorsement of the Americans with Disabilities Act Amendments Act of 2008 was signed by President Bush with additional revisions signed by the Attorney General in 2010 (ADA, 2011). There have been significant strides made in an attempt to educate all students in a fair and equitable manner. There are a multitude of disabilities that a student may have and an individual educational plan should be developed based on individual need. Furthermore, at the college and university level students must self-identify, have official documentation of the disability, and follow the policy and requirements of the organization. All faculty must comply with approved accommodations. It is important to note that the student must demonstrate the ability to complete a nursing program. There are students with and without disabilities who may not qualify for admission to a nursing program. However, the disability should not be the reason for exclusion from the program and schools legally are required to make reasonable accommodations. This chapter will present an overview of types of disabilities along with faculty and student roles and responsibilities in addition to legal issues related to educating students with disabilities.

Overview of Issue

In the past 25 years there has been a large increase in the percent of students with disabilities attending college. This trend has been evident in nursing programs with one study stating that 57.4% of nursing schools had students with learning disabilities. Traditionally, nursing educators have received limited academic preparation in teaching students with special needs (Selekman, 2002). A disability is a condition that will usually last a lifetime. Few studies have been conducted on the perceptions of faculty regarding the ability of students with disabilities to attend nursing programs. However, it is clear that some educators have serious concern as to the ability of these students. Their main concern is patient safety and fairness of accommodations. Many cannot fathom how a student in a wheelchair will be able to complete the skills necessary when caring for patients. They can't understand how a student who is hearing impaired will be able to auscultate heart and lung sounds. Students with disabilities may not be able to perform certain skills but accommodations, such as delegation of certain tasks, can be utilized (Sowers & Smith, 2004). Faculty must also be educated on the laws relating to students with disabilities. The expectation is that the student must meet the admission requirements, be able to perform the essential requirements of the program, and be given reasonable accommodations to facilitate success. Of course, this will be determined on an individualized plan as per the needs of the student. The disability may be cognitive, physical, psychological, or a combination of several different types of disabilities (Leyin, 2010).

Learning disabilities encompass a wide array of disorders that affect the way a student learns. Significant difficulties may be evident in speaking, reasoning, reading, spelling, math, and writing. "To be diagnosed with a learning disability, individuals must have at least a normal intelligence quotient, and they may even have above-normal intellectual ability. These individuals can learn they just learn differently" (Selekman, p. 334). Furthermore, students may have a physical or sensory handicap. It is important to look at each individual and make decisions based on their specific disability in regard to the requirements of the nursing program and the profession. Learning disabilities may be neurological, intellectual, or physical based and are broad spectrum so each person must be evaluated in relation to their specific needs. For example, ten students may have a diagnosis of Attention Deficit Hyperactivity Disorder but they will all have different strengths and weaknesses and require different accommodations to be successful. According to Learning Disabilities of America (LDA, 2012), learning disabilities are neurologically based and may be related to input, integration, memory, or output. For example, input may relate to visual—may see words or symbols in different order; auditory perception—may have difficulty with sound or processing of sounds; students may benefit from tape recording lectures or having someone read and explain written directions. Integration issues relate to sequencing, organization, and abstraction; students may need help with math sequencing, organizing writing assignments, and require extended testing time. Issues with memory relate to short- and long-term memory and ability to recall information; students may benefit from listening to podcasts and tape-recorded lectures and may need to break down reading assignments and learn in segments. Issues with output relate to language and motor ability; students may have difficulty expressing themselves or with fine motor skills such as writing, buttons, tying shoes, or gross motor such as walking or running. Allowing students to type their notes or use adaptive devices may be beneficial. Some well-known disabilities may be related to Attention Deficit Disorder, Dyslexia (Shellenberger, 1993), and Sensory Integration and Autism. Physical disabilities include impaired motor function, hearing, speech, and vision. Students may also have psychological issues or substance abuse issues. Psychological issues and substance abuse may be present prior to admission or emerge while the student is in the program. For example, because nursing programs are very challenging some students may become anxious or stressed and self-medicate. Or sometimes issues are not identified until young adulthood. Because each student is unique it is helpful for faculty to have a broad knowledgebase on the different types of disabilities and the types of support that are available to students. Types of support include allowing lectures to be taped, extended time on exams, use of calculators, use of computers, and organizational lists (Selekman, 2002). Faculty must also understand their role and responsibilities for students in crisis. There are confidentiality laws regarding students' personal information. However, if faculty feels the student is a danger to self or others they must follow their policy and notify the appropriate personnel. Because of confidentiality requirements faculty are usually informed only about the required accommodations and not of the specific condition. In the past students with disabilities have been discriminated against and were not seen as potential candidates in schools of nursing. Prior to the mandates of the Americans with Disabilities Act (ADA) of 1990 and Section 504 that was under the Rehabilitation Act of 1973, there were limited opportunities for students with disabilities (Jacobs & Lauber, 2011; Owen & Standen, 2007; Selekman, 2002). The ADA legislation makes it illegal to discriminate on the basis of a disability in areas of employment, public service, public accommodations, transportation, and telecommunications (Bastable, 2003, p. 281).

Educators must be aware of this law so they do not unknowingly discriminate against individuals with disabilities. Many schools and state boards of nursing have developed a list of essential skills required by nurses to use as a guideline for admission into a nursing program. However, these are guidelines and each student should be evaluated for admission into a program based on their specific needs (McCleary-Jones, 2005). Despite the laws and standards that have been passed, there remain some misconceptions about the ability of nursing students with disabilities to succeed in a nursing program (Carroll, 2004). For example, Sowers and Smith (2004) surveyed nursing faculty and found that many of them did not feel that students with disabilities could be successful in a nursing program. However, in a follow-up study, Sowers and Smith (2004) found that an educational program helped nurse educators to change their perceptions on educating students with disabilities and identified a need for continuing faculty development to ensure that decisions about individual students are based on their specific disability related to their ability to meet requirements of the nursing program and the profession. In summary, although significant strides have been made, there remains a need for faculty development in teaching students with disabilities.

Faculty Role and Responsibility

Faculty who teach in public and private institutions are obligated to follow the guidelines of the American with Disabilities Act and Section 504 in addition to being knowledgeable of the policies that govern their academic institutions. For example, if the cost and accommodations places undue burden on an institution, the institution is not obligated to accept the student into their program. Because nursing is a practice profession, issues with patient safety must also be considered. Billings and Halstead (2009) suggest that admission criteria be based on program outcomes instead of a specific set of required skills. This is an important distinction to be made because there are some technical skills that students with physical disabilities may not be able to perform but this does not mean they cannot become nurses. What it does mean is that accommodations may be required and some graduates may experience limitations as to where they can practice. Arndt (2004) identifies the qualities that every nurse needs such as caring and thinking critically, and points out the technical support can vary for some disabilities. For example, in clinical settings students may use audio-enhanced stethoscopes, electronic vital signs, assistance with lifting and positioning of patients, and be given a modified assignment. Students are not obligated to disclose their disability although some physical disabilities may be apparent during face-to-face interviews. To be eligible for accommodations, students must self-identify and supply official documentation which some students fear may negatively affect their acceptance into the program. Therefore, many students reveal their disability after they have been admitted to the program. When the student identifies and seeks support, the accommodations are developed based on the student's individual needs.

Maheady (2003) posits: "Faculty members should consider the development of an Individual Nursing Education Program for every nursing student with a disability, similar to those used with special education students in public schools" (p. 154). For example, some students require extra testing time or testing in a separate location, or the ability to record lectures. Faculty misconceptions relating to students with disabilities is predominantly due to lack of knowledge and experience with teaching students with disabilities. Many are concerned with patient safety and the ability of a student with a disability to provide safe care or that they will not be able to fulfill the requirements of their professional role. However, these concerns are often unfounded as long as appropriate support is offered. Arndt (2004) discussed how her attitude changed after reviewing different sources of literature. She learned several things about teaching a nurse with a disability. "Fairness is not achieved by treating everyone the same, but rather by giving each person what he or she needs" (Arndt, 2004, p. 205). Students with disabilities may not be able to perform certain skills but accommodations, such as delegation of certain tasks, can be utilized. "It is discriminatory to think nurses with disabilities would be any less professional in this respect than those without disabilities" (p. 206). It is recommended that educators carefully identify their own biases so they can fairly and honestly evaluate each student's performance. Some teaching strategies can be incorporated to foster learning and professional development.

Arndt (2004) recommends faculty stay current with the literature and then incorporate strategies to foster learning and professional development in support of educating nursing students with disabilities. Many accommodations can be made that benefit students with disabilities, including:

■ scribes for note taking
■ Braille examination booklets
■ large print exams
■ preferred seating
■ recorded lectures
■ extended testing time
■ testing in a separate location
■ rest periods

Because of the sparse literature on nurse faculty training related to nursing students with disabilities and the results of their previous study which demonstrated that many nurse educators do not feel qualified to teach students with disabilities, Sowers and Smith (2004) conducted a study to evaluate the efficacy of a training program on this topic. They concluded that nurses who participated in this type of training became more open to teaching students with disabilities.

Kolanko (2003) completed a collective case study to analyze the disabled nursing student's experience in baccalaureate programs. Seven students participated in the study. Five themes were identified: students had above average intelligence; instructors who were positive and organized assisted learning; families were main support; and difficulties included social isolation, anxiety, and limited time to process. Accommodations were a helpful strategy but students did not want to be labeled. Kolanko also identified strategies for faculty that included using personal stories, using knowledge in education and policy making, and utilizing knowledge of patients with neurological dysfunction in teaching students with disabilities. Addressing the issue of nursing students with physical disabilities Carroll (2004) explored the effect of including these individuals into the nursing profession. She utilized the essence of nursing as a caring, humanistic profession and articulated the theories of Roy's Adaptation Model and Watson's Caring Theory. "MacLean (1992) asserted that it is time to shift focus of nursing curricula from the technical to the humanistic. People with physical disabilities surely can deliver humanistic care to their patients" (as cited in Carroll, 2004, p. 208). Furthermore, there is a need for a "culture of inclusion" as per the ANA. Faculty attitudes rather than the physical barriers and safety concerns are a big part of the issue. In addition, nursing care for patients with disabilities could improve with the inclusion of nurses who can better empathize with their disability and conduct research relative to disabled patients. This author also found that many nursing faculty believe that students with disabilities cannot give the same level of care as non-disabled students. In contrast to this belief, she found that qualified people with disabilities are able to provide humanistic care and use their nursing knowledge to guide clinical judgment. Carroll (2004) states, "Nurse educators have a moral and ethical obligation to include them in the nursing profession so patients can benefit from their care" (p. 212). These findings support the premise that a significant percent of faculty need further education to gain a better understanding of the attributes and qualities a disabled student can bring to the profession of nursing (Carroll, 2004).

Nurse educators can take a proactive approach and continually review the literature to broaden their knowledge on educating students with special needs. They can become advocates for their students because some students with disabilities are subjected to discrimination, isolation, and rejection (Maheady, 2004). Sensitivity training and programs can be offered to faculty and students so that students with disabilities are not ostracized.

As a nurse educator you will need to be knowledgeable about the laws that relate to educating students with disabilities. Because each school has different policies you should be sure to review the policies of your school. You might want to make a general announcement to the class about the policy for self-disclosure and the procedure to follow to apply for accommodations. You will receive an official notification from your school about the specific accommodations your students have been granted. You will need to work with your students and administrators to ensure that all accommodations are met. For example, if a student requires extended testing time or testing in a separate location you will need to make arrangements prior to the day of the exam and inform the student of the arrangements. Confidentiality must be maintained to protect the rights of students. You do not have the right to question students about their specific disability, only the accommodations. However, at times this may be challenging because other students may be aware when one or two students are not part of the class during exams or have to use assistive devices. But as long as you do not disclose the information it is up to the individual student if they decide to tell faculty and students about their disability. Faculty and academic organizations may be sued if they discriminate against students with disabilities in regards to admission and accommodations so it is vital to adhere to the policies (Billings & Halstead, 2009). The most important thing is to be supportive and serve as an advocate for all students and to seek guidance from school administrators whenever you need clarification or support.

Faculty from the University of Manitoba shared their experience in educating students with disabilities. Throughout the process there were challenges that had to be faced but they found that by decreasing barriers and offering support, students could be successful. Furthermore, conducting a self-examination and delineating clear roles and responsibilities was beneficial to all. At times faculty must leave their comfort zone and think out of the box to develop strategies to foster success in students with disabilities because students with disabilities who have the intellectual ability and willingness to learn can thrive in a supportive environment (Ashcroft et al., 2008). In summary, the American Disabilities Act and Section 504 of the Rehabilitation Act of 1973 protect the rights of all people with disabilities. However, it does not guarantee admission into all programs as the individual must have the potential to succeed with support. Furthermore, although academic organizations must provide reasonable accommodations, they must not place undue financial burden on the organization.

Student Role and Responsibility

Nursing students with disabilities must learn how to advocate for themselves and address the challenges and strategies to overcome obstacles. Students are advised to inform nursing programs of accommodations required. Although some students may be hesitant to reveal they have a disability, they will not be given accommodations unless they self-identify and follow the procedures set forth in their colleges and universities. In the past, some educators have been concerned about the type of nursing students with disabilities can perform; however, there are multiple areas for nurses with disabilities to work. They include: home care, case management, parish nurse, research, and a host of other areas (Evans, 2005; Maheady, 1999).

There are many organizations that have been created to address the special needs of students and nurses with all types of disabilities. Exceptionalnurse. com is a resource network that offers multiple resources and information to nurses with disabilities. The organization is also committed to increasing the number of people with disabilities into the nursing profession. The National Organization of Nurses with Disabilities (NOND, 2012) is another organization that offers advocacy and support to nurses with disabilities and chronic health conditions. According to their website their goal is to provide resources, and to promote best practices and equity among nurses with disabilities. The National Student Nurse Association recently supported a resolution that was presented by the Georgia Student Nurses Association on the education of students with disabilities. The resolution *Promoting a Positive Image of Nursing Students with Disabilities* addressed the issue of students with disabilities and calls for the fair and equitable treatment of students with disabilities. Furthermore, they plan to spotlight nursing students with disabilities and publish articles. They are also planning to share this with the following agencies: the National Council of State Boards, the American Nurses Association, the National League for Nursing, the National Organization for Associate Degree Nursing, the American Association of Colleges of Nursing, the National Organization of Nurses with Disabilities, and Minority Nurse (National Student Nurses Association, 2011).

DISABILITIES AND CULTURAL COMPETENCE

The issue of nursing students with disabilities and cultural competence was explored by Marks (2007). The purpose of the paper was to demonstrate how increasing the recruitment of nursing students can augment culturally competent care. The author discussed the importance of inclusion and understanding of disabilities. Utilizing the social model and the minority group model identifies a disability as a social status rather than a physical or cognitive attribute. Many people with disabilities feel that the way people react to them is harder than dealing with their disability. This is due to lack of understanding on the part of healthcare professionals, which creates a cultural conflict. This results in discrimination of care based on disability status, which is known as ableist. The author makes several valid points in regard to education, incorporation of the social model of disability, acceptance of people with disabilities, and accommodations for nursing students with disabilities. Furthermore, acceptance of students with disabilities will enhance culturally competent nursing care. This article raised valid issues that should be investigated further with a formal research study (Marks, 2007).

EXEMPLAR

A nursing student who had a physical disability that required the use of a wheelchair and a canine companion was admitted to a nursing program in Washington and the response to this by the faculty ranged from shock and discomfort to acceptance and a willingness to participate in this new educational journey. According to Evans (2005), Victoria was one of the first wheelchair bound students to graduate, obtain licensure, and practice as Registered Nurse in the United States. Evans (2005), who was the instructor assigned to this student, shared her journey in the hopes that nurse faculty will realize the importance of inclusion and social justice for people with disabilities. Evans points out that the student had the intellectual ability to become a nurse and that according to the National Council of the State Boards of Nursing there are eight functional ability groups for nurses to practice, which include fine motor skills, hearing, arithmetic competence, emotional stability, analytical thinking, critical thinking, interpersonal skills, and communication skills. She noted that walking was not on the list and therefore they had to provide a "reasonable accommodation" while maintaining the standards of the curriculum. It is often difficult to conceptualize how a student with a disability can be a nurse but the story of Victoria and her instructor clearly demonstrates that students with disabilities who are given support can be successful in a nursing program (Evans, 2005).

SUMMARY

This chapter focused on educating nursing students with disabilities. Legal issues were discussed in relation to admission and student accommodations. An overview of disabilities and potential student accommodations was also presented.

DISCUSSION QUESTIONS

1. Discuss the legal issues surrounding the admission and education of students with disabilities.
2. List three types of disabilities and accommodation strategies.
3. Describe the role of faculty in educating students with disabilities.
4. Describe the role of the student in self-disclosure.
5. Discuss your personal feelings on the ability of students with disabilities to complete a nursing program.

SUGGESTED LEARNING ACTIVITIES

- Interview a faculty member about his/her perspective of nursing students with disabilities.
- Compare and contrast the admission policies at three different schools on admission criteria for students with disabilities.
- Interview a nurse with a disability and write an essay about his or her experience as a student and a nurse.

Creating a Welcome Mat for Nursing Students With Disabilities

DONNA CAROL MAHEADY, EdD, ARNP

TEACHING NURSING STUDENTS WITH DISABILITIES BRINGS to mind Bob Dylan's song "The times they are a-changin'." In the past, student with disabilities were denied admission to nursing programs. In reality some were admitted—but scared silent in fear of rejection or dismissal. Fortunately, nursing students with disabilities can now openly disclose a disability—if willing—and receive reasonable accommodations. I am often asked, "Has the tide from earlier decades turned in support of nursing students with disabilities?" Based on over 10 years of work as an advocate for nurses and nursing students with disabilities, the tide hasn't turned completely. At some colleges and universities, the gains have been substantial. In other programs, there has barely been a ripple. Much depends on the attitude of faculty and administrators. The positive news is that more and more students with a wide range of disabilities are being admitted, progressing, and graduating from nursing programs. The Americans with Disabilities Act and a generally more positive attitude toward people with disabilities have helped to pave the way.

You will be guiding the next generation of nursing students including those with disabilities. You may be saying to yourself ...."but I'm not prepared," "where can I turn for help"? or "what can I do to welcome students with disabilities"? The following suggestions will help you create a solid welcome mat.

Build on Your Previous Skills and Experiences

You know more than you think. Remember all of the patients you helped to navigate the healthcare system and adjust to disability and other health concerns. Now, a similar person is no longer your patient—but your student.

Make Friends With the Disabilities Services Office

The Disabilities Services office is an important resource for faculty and students. Disabilities Services staff will formulate an accommodation plan and provide needed supports such as note takers, sign language interpreters, and audio books.

Keep an Open Mind and Think Outside of the Box

Students with disabilities bring unique abilities to nursing. Often, they have been patients on the receiving end of care—where the seeds for a career in nursing were planted when they were cared for by a nurse who had an impact on their life. Through personal experience, they may have developed remarkable compensatory abilities and insight into the needs of patients. Some have been struggling for years to land in your classroom or clinical group.

Know Your Legal Obligations as Well as the Student's Rights to Reasonable Accommodations

The Americans with Disabilities Act was passed in 1990 and amended in 2008 in an effort to level the playing field for people with disabilities. Familiarity with the law will benefit you and your student.

Serve as an Acceptance Bridge

Fellow students may view reasonable accommodations received by a student with a disability as lowering the bar or unfair advantage. Be prepared for possible negative comments or attitudes.

Recognize That Reasonable Accommodations Are a Floor Not a Ceiling

Patience, acceptance, and understanding from you will go a long way in facilitating a student's success. In addition a positive attitude—and serving as an acceptance bridge—will influence other faculty members, students, patients, and clinical agency staff. Students with disabilities may require a longer amount of time to learn new skills and may perform skills in a different way.

Clinical Experiences

Whenever possible, try to meet with the student with a disability prior to the start of a clinical rotation. The more familiar you are with the student and his or her accommodation plan—the better.

Familiarize Yourself With Resources Available to Assist Faculty and Students

When confronted with a student with disability or chronic illness, recognize that you are most likely not the first faculty member to work with a similarly situated student. Reach out to organizations that assist nurses and nursing students with disabilities—where you can find answers to questions like "Where can a student find an appropriate amplified stethoscope?" "Are gloves made for nurses with missing fingers?" "How can a nurse with one hand start an IV?" "How can a nurse who uses a wheelchair perform CPR?" Link up with a veteran nursing faculty member who can offer guidance and share best practices. Encourage the student to get involved with organizations and find a mentor with a similar challenge. Search the nursing literature for articles and books written about nursing students with disabilities. Groups are on social media (Facebook, Twitter) as well.

NCLEX

Be aware of your state board of nursing's policy related to requests for reasonable accommodations. Advise your student to be aware as well. Applications need to be submitted early and include required documentation.

Accommodations Level the Playing Field, But Aren't a Guarantee of Success

Students with disabilities should be held to the same standards as other students. One of the most difficult challenges of being a nurse educator is recognizing that not every student (disabled or nondisabled) will be successful in a nursing program. Keep the bar high for all students!

As a new faculty member you can be the face and voice of change. Disability is part of life for all of us. Students with disabilities can enrich the nursing profession and add value to health care. An open mind and positive attitude will do much to dispel the myth that every nurse has to have a strong back and perfect hearing and vision. When you receive your first or next notification regarding an accommodation plan for a nursing student, instead of thinking, "No way," think "Why not"? An attitude that celebrates the gifts that all students can bring to nursing will shine on your classroom or clinical group and benefit everyone. Through your students, you will be taught!

REFERENCES

Arndt, M. (2004). Educating nursing students with disabilities: One nurse educator's journey questions to clarity. *Journal of Nursing Education, 43*(5), 204–206.

Ashcroft, T., Chernomas, W., Davis, P., Dean, R., Seguire, M., Shapiro, C., & Swiderski, L. (2008). Nursing students with disabilities: One faculty's journey. *International Journal of Nursing Education Scholarship, 5*(1), 1–15.

ADA Home Page—ada.gov—Information and Technical Assistance. Retrieved from www.ada.gov/

Bastable, S. (2003). *Nurse as educator principles of teaching and learning for nurse practice* (2nd ed.). Sudbury, MA: Jones & Bartlett.

Billings, D. M., & Halstead, J. A. (2009). Teaching in nursing: A guide for faculty (3rd ed.). Philadelphia, PA: W.B. Saunders.

Carroll, S. (2004). Inclusion of people with physical disabilities in nursing education. *Journal of Nursing Education, 43*(5), 207–212.

Evans, B. C. (2005). Nursing education for students with disabilities: Our students, our teachers. *Annual Review of Nursing Education, 3*, 1.

Jacobs, R. B., & Lauber, R. H. (2011). Realities of the Americans with Disabilities Act. *Employee Relations Law Journal, 37*(1), 35–59.

Kolanko K. (2003). A collective case study of nursing students with learning disabilities. *Nursing Education Perspectives, 24*(5), 251–256.

Learning Disabilities Association of America. (2012). *Types of learning disabilities.* Retrieved from www.ldanatl.org/aboutld/teachers/understanding/types.asp

Leyin, A. (2010). Learning disability classification: time for re-appraisal? *Tizard Learning Disability Review, 15*(2), 33–44.

Maheady, D. (1999). Jumping through hoops, walking on egg shells: The experiences of nursing students with disabilities. *Journal of Nursing Education, 38*(4), 162–170.

Maheady, D. (2003). *Nursing students with disabilities change the course.* River Edge, NJ: Exceptional Parent Press.

Marks, B. (2007). Cultural competence revisited: nursing students with disabilities. *Journal of Nursing Education, 46*(2), 70–74.

McCleary-Jones, V. (2005). The Americans with Disabilities Act of 1990 and its impact on higher education and nursing education. *ABNF Journal, 16*(2), 24–27.

National Organization of Nurses with Disabilities (NOND). (2012). NOND is an open membership, cross-disability, professional organization that works to promote equity for people with disabilities and chronic health conditions in nursing. Retrieved from www.nond.org.

National Student Nurses Association. Resolution on Nursing Students with Disabilities. (2011). Retrieved from www.nsna.org/Portals/0/Skins/NSNA/pdf/pubs_guide_resolutions.pdf

Owen, S., & Standen, P. (2007). Attracting and retaining learning disability student nurses. *British Journal of Learning Disabilities, 35*(4), 261–268.

Selekman, J. (2002). Nursing students with disabilities. *Journal of Nursing Education, 41*(8), 334–340.

Shellenberger, T. (1993). Helping dyslexic nursing students. *Nurse Educator, 18*(6), 10–13.

Sowers, J., & Smith, M. (2004). Evaluation of the effects of an inservice training program on nursing faculty members' perceptions, knowledge, and concerns about students with disabilities. *Journal of Nursing Education, 43*(6), 248–252.

FURTHER READINGS

Dupler, A., Allen, C., Maheady, D., Fleming, S., & Allen, M. (2012). Leveling the playing field for nursing students with disabilities: Implications of the Amendments to the Americans with Disabilities Act. *Journal of Nursing Education, 51*(3), 140–144.

http://www.washington.edu/doit/ DO-IT Center promotes the success of individuals with disabilities in postsecondary education and careers, using technology as an empowering tool.

Maheady, D. (2003). *Nursing students with disabilities change the course.* River Edge, NJ: Exceptional Parent Press.

Maheady, D. C. (2005). Teaching nursing students with disabilities. In L. Caputi (Ed.), *Teaching nursing: The art and science* (Vol. 3, pp. 209–231). Glen Ellyn, IL: College of DuPage Press.

Maheady, D. C. (2006). *Leave no nurse behind: Nurses working with disabilities.* Lincoln, NE: iUniverse, Inc.

Righting the Americans with Disabilities National Council on Disabilities (2004). Retrieved from www.ncd.gov/publications/2004.org

The National Joint Committee on Learning Disabilities. (2011). Comprehensive assessment and evaluation of students with learning disabilities. *Learning Disability Quarterly, 34*(1), 3–16.

www.amphl.org The Association of Medical Professionals with Hearing Losses is a network for individuals with hearing loss interested in or working in health care fields.

www.ExceptionalNurse.com ExceptionalNurse.com is a non-profit resource network for nurses and nursing students with disabilities.

www.Learningally.org Learning ally provides accessible learning materials for students with visual or learning disabilities.

CHAPTER 20

Reflective Journaling

"By three methods we may learn wisdom: First, by reflection, which is noblest; second, by imitation, which is easiest; and third by experience, which is the bitterest."

—CONFUCIUS

OBJECTIVES

After reading this chapter, the reader will be able to
- Understand the importance of journaling for self-development
- Discuss the use of reflective journaling in the classroom
- Identify key components of a journal
- Understand emotional intelligence
- Compare and contrast journaling and narrative pedagogy

INTRODUCTION

The benefits of journaling in nursing and other fields have been well documented (Charles, 2010; Fritson, Forrest, & Bohl, 2011). According to Hiemstra (2001) journals may include insights, personal thoughts, and experiences. Journaling is a process by which a person engages in self-reflection through written accounts of positive and negative personal experiences. Through the process of critical self-reflection a person may reflect on the meaning of what has been learned and expand their worldview. This type of activity may help to relieve stress and guide the person in the continued holistic development of self (Scott, 2011). Journaling has been utilized in undergraduate and graduate nursing programs to help students develop critical thinking and personal development (Charles, 2010). In this chapter the use of journaling for self-development in addition to the use of journaling for student development will be presented. The key components of journaling will also be discussed however, because personal journaling is a unique experience for the individual there is no definitive way to keep a journal. Nevertheless, when utilizing journaling as a teaching and learning strategy, faculty may assign formal or informal journals.

JOURNALING FOR SELF-DEVELOPMENT

Journaling is the process of writing down one's lived experiences. The purpose and intent of journaling is done for many different reasons. For example, some nursing students keep journals because it is a requirement of their course. Many people keep a journal as a means to partake in the act of self-reflection. Writers keep journals to write down snippets or ideas for future story ideas. Many people keep journals to document their academic or professional journey. Evers (2008) states that journaling can be a way to put something to rest as one can let go of problems by writing them in a journal. For some there may be a spiritual element where they meditate or pray through their journaling. It may also be used as a catharsis by writing down negative events or feelings. Journaling may also be used for self-development. Smith (2009) discusses the relationship of narrative journaling and emotional intelligence. Emotional intelligence relates to non-cognitive skills and has been associated with the ability to become successful in one's life. Indeed, successful individuals need to have both emotional intelligence and cognitive intelligence (Freshwater & Stickley, 2004). The inclusion of emotional intelligence in nursing has become increasingly popular and Freshwater and Stickley (2004) recommend that it be included in all the nursing curriculums. They suggest the following examples of what should be included in the curriculum: reflective learning, self-inquiry, narrative, and mentorship. "Conceptualized by two psychologists, Salovey and Mayer's, they define emotional intelligence as being able to monitor and regulate one's own feelings, understand the feelings of other's and use that 'feeling' knowledge to guide thoughts and actions" (Smith, 2009, p. 84). Journaling in this respect is an activity that allows for reflection and integration of the experience which in turn helps the person to develop critical thinking skills. Although this study focused on student development it also has applicability for the nurse educator. It is very helpful to write down one's thoughts and feelings in regard to your academic journey. Reflecting on one's personal journey is an important step in self-development and the continued development of emotional intelligence. The transition from clinician to academic may be a smooth path for some and a bumpy road for others. Journaling can help you to analyze your experiences and let go of some of the stress and negativity. Furthermore, when you look back at an event you can usually look at it more objectively, which helps you to be more realistic. A problem that seemed major at the time it occurred may be viewed differently after some time has elapsed. Reflecting on areas you have excelled in and areas for improvement helps you continue your personal and professional development. Sometimes you are so busy with day-to-day activities that you do not realize how much you have accomplished over six months or a year. However, if you have kept a journal you can actually see how you have developed. This can also be helpful when applying for promotion and tenure as you will have a written account of the various activities of teaching, service, and scholarship. Osterman and Kottkamp (1993) discuss reflective practice and self-awareness in faculty. They posit that faculty who engage in reflective practice have a dual role and use the analogy of the actor and the critic. On one hand the educator is immersed in their role similar to an actor and on the other hand the educator can analyze their performance much like a critic. By doing this the faculty member can become more aware of their actions and behaviors which may have a positive impact on personal growth and development. Stress reduction is another benefit of journaling. Although there are many ways to partake in the practice of keeping a journal, the act itself can help you to become grounded and as you write you may notice that you are becoming less tense. Keeping a journal also helps you develop writing skills because your thoughts will be flowing, and as you place your words on paper or type them into a Word document, you become totally immersed in your task. It is a very personal experience and can be done in any format wherever and whenever you have the desire to journal. Although scholarly writing is a more formal process than writing in a journal, journaling does help you to develop as a writer because all types of writing are beneficial. The adage to be a writer you must write is very true. In summary, keeping a journal has personal and professional benefits.

JOURNALING AND STUDENT DEVELOPMENT

The use of reflective journaling (Blake, 2005), and narrative pedagogy (Brown, Kirkpatrick, Mangum, & Avery, 2009), has been embraced by many nurse educators in undergraduate and graduate programs in an attempt to enhance critical thinking, self-awareness, and self-development (Grendell, 2011). Students may be required to journal formally with specific guidelines, or informally with freedom to develop their own journal. Reflective journaling often involves a more formal process and faculty may provide specific guidelines for students to follow. Many students prefer guidelines especially if they have never kept a journal. Providing clear guidelines can help to allay their fears in the process of journaling (Epp, 2008).

Narrative pedagogy is somewhat similar yet different than journaling (Nehls, 1995). Grendell (2011) describes narrative pedagogy as interpretive and something that requires in-depth analysis of a situation that promotes discovery and problem-solving—for example, a clinical experience. "Narrative pedagogy can enhance research-based curricula, especially through use of innovative technologies that promote holistic thinking and problem solving, to prepare nursing students for the complexity of the profession" (Grendell, 2011, p. 66). Because narrative pedagogy may promote critical thinking and reasoning it has great applicability in nursing programs. Ironside (2006) conducted a hermeneutic study on student's experiences in courses where teachers utilized narrative pedagogy. Ironside describes narrative pedagogy as "community interpretive scholarship" which brings together phenomenology, critical theory, post-modern theory, and feminist theories. She concluded that utilizing this type of pedagogy encourages students to think and interpret and create multiple perspectives on situations. As faculties understand the limitations of traditional pedagogies they are beginning to embrace narrative pedagogy as a means to enhance the development of critical reasoning and thinking in their students. Kirkpatrick and Brown (2004) posit that a paradigm shift in utilizing narrative pedagogy—a humanistic approach for reflection and critical thinking entails a shared reflection and interpretation between faculty and student. This pedagogy is recognized as an innovative method for fostering a collaborative learning environment. Kirkpatrick and Brown (2004) demonstrate how this pedagogy can be applied in a geriatric course through the use of stories and reflection. Listening to and reflecting upon the stories of the geriatric patients helped students and patients to develop therapeutic relationships. Narrative pedagogy is becoming increasingly popular and may be used in a variety of courses. It is especially beneficial in theory/clinical courses and helps students to develop critical thinking and reasoning skills, problem solving, and holistic care.

Blake (2005) completed a review of the literature on journaling and noted that although journaling is widely embraced there have been few quantitative studies. Although there were more qualitative than quantitative studies, further research is warranted. Blake identified several benefits of journaling, which include discovering meaning of an experience; making connections between theory and practice; instilling values such as altruism; understanding perspectives of patients; reflecting on nursing role; improving writing and critical thinking skills; developing affective skills such as empathy; and the ability to care for oneself in response to human suffering (p. 7). Lauterbach and Hentz (2005) describe journaling as a way to enhance self-reflection in nursing students. This is probably one of the most beneficial aspects of journaling, especially in nursing. The nature of nursing is one where nurses deal with a myriad of personal and patient emotions. They may be witnessing the miracle of birth or holding a patient's hand as they are in the process of dying. One day may be filled with joy and the next filled with grief. When students have an opportunity to write down their experiences and then reflect upon them, it can help to put things in perspective. "As an educational process, refection facilitates students' leaning to identify, discover, explicate, and develop the requisite knowledge and values that will provide the foundation for their practice" (Lauterbach & Hentz, 2005 p. 31). Because of the complexity of nursing practice students who journal can synthesize and integrate knowledge and apply it in the care of their patients. Many of us reflect on our experiences even if we don't journal but journaling offers a broader dimension of reflection. At first students may not embrace journaling but once they become comfortable with the process most of them will realize the benefits and continue to journal throughout their nursing careers. Lauterbach and Hentz (2005) recommend that students and faculty alike develop a habit of journaling as frequent journaling and reflection will help the person to become more reflective and improve critical thinking. Students should be comfortable with the process and share only the information they feel comfortable sharing with others. Of course, there are many ways to journal and this will be discussed in the next section. However, students need some type of guideline for their journal and faculty should support students as they engage in this process. They should also be assured that their journals are confidential and that they will not be shared with others unless they give permission. For example, sometimes during post-conference the students may share snippets of information that were especially meaningful to them. However, they may choose not to share their innermost feelings on the topic. Therefore, faculty has the responsibility to protect their students when reading journals and be careful not to violate their rights to privacy and confidentiality. This might be accomplished by having students reflect on their journals and write a brief summary of what they would like to share with you and perhaps their fellow students. Students should feel comfortable when writing in their journals and be able to choose what they wish to share. Waldo and Hermanns (2009) discuss how journaling can be used to address fears during the psychiatric clinical experience. Beginning in 2007 they piloted a program where students would journal and also partake in some form of creative expression. The students are given specific instructions and have the option of sharing their creative work. To date they have piloted this activity for five semesters and there results have been positive. The students consider this to be a valuable experience that has helped them to provide holistic care, think critically, and deal with stressful situations. Van Horn and Freed (2008) investigated the use of journaling and dialogue pairs in 39 nursing students who were in a clinical course. They found that the combination of working in pairs and journaling led to increased reflection and was beneficial to both students. This is a new approach and the authors noted that there were no other studies found on this topic. However, the results of this study support it as teaching strategy that warrants further evaluation. In summary, journaling, narrative pedagogy, and reflective practice should be included and threaded throughout the curriculum. Benefits of these activities include self-reflection, development of critical thinking and reasoning skills, integration of theory and clinical, stress reduction, and growth and development. Partaking in these pedagogies may also help individuals to develop emotional intelligence which has been linked to successful people. There are many ways to engage in journaling and narrative pedagogy and it is important to be clear about your expectations and maintain confidentiality in addition to protecting the student's right to privacy.

WAYS TO JOURNAL

Journaling can be done in many different ways and there is no right or wrong way to journal. Journals may be structured or unstructured. Journal assignments may have specific guidelines and grading rubrics. Or they may have broad guidelines with pass/fail grades. Sometimes faculties recommend that students keep a personal journey but do not make it a mandatory assignment. In this type of journal the students just write at will whenever they feel like writing and they do not share their reflections with anyone. As a nurse educator you will need to consider several factors before you develop your assignment, for example:

- What course objective does this assignment evaluate?
- Will it be a structured assignment?
- Will it be graded?
- Will students be required to share a summary of their journals?
- What is the purpose of this assignment?
    - *Integrating theoretical and clinical concepts*
    - *Narrative pedagogy*
    - *Self-evaluation*
    - *Professional development*
    - *Reflection*
    - *Development of critical thinking and reasoning skills*
    - *Stress reduction*
- How many journal entries will the student be assigned?
- What percent of the course grade will be allocated?

Developing an assignment takes time and planning. Thinking about the purpose and intent of your assignment will help you to create an assignment that is relevant to your course.

It is important to review the literature and sample assignments that can be tailored to meet your needs. Because evidence-based evaluation is important you will want to measure the effectiveness of your assignment in achieving your goals. It is a good idea to pilot an assignment and revise it as necessary. Fritson, Forrest, and Bohl (2011) recommend keeping the journal impersonal so as not to cause discomfort. If you feel it will be beneficial to have students write down negative events and feelings you may limit what they will have to share. Deciding how much or how often you expect students to journal is another area to consider. Fritson et al. (2011) suggest that if the journals are being grading the faculty should consider their ability to grade journals in a timely fashion and to consider the workload of the student. Journals, whether structured or unstructured, formal or informal, graded or ungraded, are beneficial in the academic and personal lives of faculty and students. Fritson et al. (2011) posit: "The learning relationship becomes more reciprocal and students become more reflective of both the course material and how to best learn that course material" (p. 160). The art and science of journaling takes time to cultivate in students but once the foundation is set many students continue to journal even when it is not a course requirement. Engaging in journaling has many positive benefits and should be considered as a teaching and learning strategy, especially in clinical courses. There are many ways to incorporate journaling into your courses so be creative, think out of the box, and be sure to relate your assignment to the curriculum and course objectives.

SUMMARY

Journaling has many benefits and can be used across the curriculum. Journaling may be done for personal or professional growth. Both faculty and students may engage in journaling which may help them improve emotional intelligence, critical thinking and reasoning skills, and problem solving. Additional benefits include self-reflection, self-evaluation, and stress reduction. When faculty is using journaling as a formal means of teaching and evaluation, they should consider the overall goals of the assignment (see sample assignment at end of chapter).

DISCUSSION QUESTIONS

1. What are the personal benefits of journaling?
2. Compare and contrast narrative pedagogy and journaling.
3. Describe emotional intelligence.
4. What are the potential negative effects of journaling?
5. What is the difference between a structured and unstructured journal?

SUGGESTED LEARNING ACTIVITIES

- Keep a journal for three months and reflect on the process.
- Review the literature and develop a journaling assignment for a course of your choice.
- Interview two faculty members about their use of narrative pedagogy and/ or reflective journaling.

SAMPLE ASSIGNMENT—MEDICAL-SURGICAL CLINICAL

Narrative Pedagogy (10%)

Describe:

- the clinical situation (patient, staff, environment)
- your situation with the patient
- your concerns at the time
- QSEN competencies in relation to your situation

Reflect:

- your thoughts as the situation was unfolding
- your feelings during and after the situation
- what was the most challenging; most rewarding
- important conversations you had with the patient, family, staff, and others
- what you would have done differently
- other important factors

Discuss:

- share this reflection with group[1]
- current analysis of situation
- lessons learned

REFERENCES

Brown, Kirkpatrick, Mangum, & Avery. (2008). A review of narrative pedagogy strategies to transform traditional nursing education. *Journal of Nursing Education, 47*(6):283–286.

Blake, T. (2005). Journaling: An active learning technique. *International Journal of Nursing Education Scholarship, 2*(1)(7), 1–13.

Brown, S., Kirkpatrick, M., Greer, A., Matthias, A., & Swanson, M. (2009). The use of innovative pedagogies in nursing education: An international perspective. *Nursing Education Perspectives, 30*(3), 153–158.

Charles, J. (2010). Journaling: Creating space for "i." *Creative Nursing, 16*(4), 180–184. doi: 10.1891/1078-4535.16.4.180

Epp, S. (2008). The value of reflective journaling in undergraduate nursing education: A literature review. *International Journal of Nursing Studies, 45*(9), 1379–1388. doi: 10.1016/j.ijnurstu.2008.01.006

Evers, F. T. (2008). Journaling: A path to our innermost self. *Interbeing, 2*(2), 53–56.

Freshwater, D., & Stickley, T. (2004). The heart of the art: Emotional intelligence in nurse education. *Nursing Inquiry, 11*(2), 91–98.

Fritson, K. K., Forrest, K. D., & Bohl, M. L. (2011). *Using reflective journaling in the college course.* Dubuque, IA: APA Division 2, Society for the Teaching of Psychology.

Grendell, R. N. (2011). Narrative pedagogy, technology, and curriculum transformation in nursing education. *Journal of Leadership Studies, 4*(4), 65–67. doi: 10.1002/jls.20197

Hiemstra, R. (2001). Uses and benefits of journal writing. In L. M. English & M. A. Gillen, (Eds.), *Promoting journal writing in adult education* (New Directions for Adult and Continuing Education, No. 90, pp. 19–26). San Francisco, CA: Jossey-Bass.

Ironside, P. M. (2006). Using narrative pedagogy: Learning and practising interpretive thinking. *Journal of Advanced Nursing, 55*(4), 478–486. doi: 10.1111/j.1365-2648.2006.03938.x

Kirkpatrick, M., & Brown, S. (2004). Narrative pedagogy: Teaching geriatric content with stories and the "Make a Difference" Project (MADP). *Nursing Education Perspectives, 25*(4), 183–187.

---

[1]Only share what you are comfortable sharing with the group.

Lauterbach, S., & Hentz, P. (2005). Journaling to learn: A strategy in nursing education for developing the nurse as person and person as nurse. *International Journal for Human Caring, 9*(1), 29–35.

Nehls, N. (1995). Narrative pedagogy: Rethinking nursing education. *Journal of Nursing Education, 34*, 204–210.

Osterman, A., & Kottkamp, R. (1993). *Reflective practice for educators improving schooling through professional development.* Newbury Park, CA: Corwin Press Inc.

Scott, E. (2011). The benefits of journaling for stress management. *About.com Guide.* Retrieved from http://www.about.com

Smith, J. (2009). Emotional intelligence and professional education: The use of narrative journaling. *International Journal of Learning, 16*(7), 81–92.

Van Horn, R., & Freed, S. (2008). Journaling and dialogue pairs to promote reflection in clinical nursing education. *Nursing Education Perspectives, 29*(4), 220–225.

Waldo, N., & Hermanns, M. (2009). Journaling unlocks fears in clinical practice. *RN, 72*(5), 26–31.

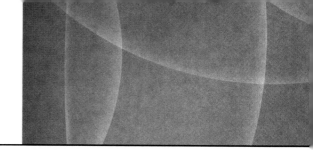

Index